Natural
Healing
Handbook

Get back to health
...Naturally!

By Beth M. Ley

Foreword by Dr. Arnold J. Susser, R.P. Ph.D.

This book is not intended to serve as medical advice. Its intention is solely information and educational. Quantities shown for beneficial supplementation are not prescriptive. Some dosages are high and represent therapeutic test dosages. Individual needs and tolerances will vary according to body size, metabolism, age, diet and ailment. Please consult a medical or health professional should the need for one be warranted.

NOTE: Mega doses of certain nutrients for prolonged periods, such as vitamin A, are not recommended unless one is under a doctor's supervision. Harmful levels may buildup in the body if high dosages are taken for prolonged periods.

BL Publications
1638 Westcliff Drive
Newport Beach, CA 92660
714-645-9718

Printed in the United States of America

Credits:
Assistance in Editing and Cover Design:
Lisa Habbeshaw

TABLE OF CONTENTS

FOREWORD

I have not always known the value of natural healing. I spent much of my early adult life involved in the orthodox allopathic field of medicine as a pharmacist and as a medical detail man for a major pharmaceutical firm. My responsibility was to call on physicians, inform and instruct them on the benefits, dosages and side effects of the drugs sold through my company. We manufactured and sold every type of drug possible for conditions ranging from mental illness to fungus of the toe.

In the course of my 17-plus years in the field, I called on nearly 40,000 medical doctors. I shared the opinion with my physician contacts that if you could not treat a symptom, then you just might have to "cut it out." With the pharmaceutical education I had, I simply thought that drugs and surgery were the cure for everything. I did not know the area of natural medicine even existed.

Later through an illness of my own and wanting to avoid mastoid surgery, I fell into the area of natural healing. Low and behold it worked! It was then that I discovered there was something else out there and I decided to go back to school and became totally involved in natural health.

In 1972 I remember feeling secure in my vast amount of knowledge about health and medicine. Now 18 years later I realize what I knew was drugs, and I knew very little about natural health. Now I realize how much more I have learned and how much expertise there is out there. It is ironic how at a certain age we seem to feel that we know a lot, and then five or ten years later we realize how little we actually did know. As life goes on we learn more and more everyday.

Although I have a vast experience in my research of books, newsletters, periodicals and publications throughout the health field, it was with great pleasure that I accepted this invitation to write the Foreword to this book and join the notable company of contributors to this book.

Three cheers!
Make that 77-plus cheers for Beth M. Ley and the "Natural Healing Handbook!"

The author has successfully and brilliantly expanded the standard 26-letter alphabet to a 77-plus-letter alphabet of extremely valuable health information and guidance.

After a thorough, but "easy-to-digest" Part I on nutrition, Beth moves on in Part II to a clearly presented discussion of no less than 77 ailments and conditions of health in an easy-to-follow alphabetical order. Her expert style and handling of this and other subject matter through this book is done with both uniqueness and originality of thought as well as consideration for the reader.

"Natural Healing Handbook" exhibits true meaning to the phrase, "Health is Wealth." This book contains a wealth of knowledge contributed virtually by a "Who's Who" in the health and nutrition field, presented in an easy to read, enjoyable format.

The reader benefits from the expertise from a highly respected and distinguished group of individuals including renowned researcher and chemist Dr. Jeffrey Bland, President of HealthComm, Inc., and former director of the Nutritional Supplement Analysis Laboratory at the Linus Pauling Institute of Science and Medicine; Dr. Linus Pauling, himself, nobel prize winner noted as "the greatest chemist of the 20th century," and for his work with vitamin C; Dr. Stephen Levine, for his work with allergies, chemical sensitivities and free radicals; Dr. Keith Sehnert, known for his work with Candida-Related Complex (CRC), the immune system, medical self-care, nutrition, and stress management; Dr. John Willard, creator of the patented Catalyst Altered Water; Dr. Hal Huggins, known for his work on mercury (dental fillings) related toxic diseases; Dr. Paul Eck, noted scientist and mineral researcher; Dr. William McGarey, noted physician for his work with the body, mind and spirit, and work with castor oil, Dr. Oscar Rasmussen, renowned nutritionist; Michael Tierra, noted outstanding herbalist; Udo Erasmus, prominent authority on the subject of fats and oils.

This book is truly the wealthiest source of health and nutrition information ever compiled in a single publication. Just a glance at the introduction, index, appendix, and bibliography will give the reader an exciting sense of awareness of what this book has to offer. This book gives a positive hope to the improvement of one's life without drugs

This book covers every possible ailment or condition that I have seen in my practice, plus a few others. "Natural Healing Handbook" can serve as a valuable usable reference book for years to come!

Whether you want to stay in good health or get back to good health naturally, this book belongs in your "Health is Wealth" library. "Natural Healing Handbook" truly offers something for everyone!

Dr. Arnold Susser

Dr. Arnold Susser, President of Great Life Labs, is a registered pharmacist, has a Ph.D. in nutrition and is a licensed naturopathic physician. He is the nutritional consultant to the trainers of the San Francisco Giants and the New York Yankees. In addition, he is the founder of the American Academy of Nutritional Consultants, the Nutrition Society of America, and is the author of the book, "The Indigestion of America From Headaches to Hemorrhoids."

INTRODUCTION

This guidebook was designed to provide useful information about ways to improve one's health and well being through natural means. Education about what good health is and what the body needs to obtain and maintain good health is important so that we can make the best decisions for ourselves.

Good health should not be thought of as absence of disease. We should avoid negative disease-orientated thinking and try to concentrate on what we have to do to remain healthy. Health is maintaining on a daily basis what is essential to the body while disease is the result of attempting to live without what the body needs. We are responsible for our own health, and should get in control of it. If we are in control of our health, disease will not take control.

Our health depends on education.

Natural Healing

The purpose of natural healing is to remove the cause of disease without harmful drugs or unnecessary surgery. Natural healing utilizes natural therapies including nutrition (vitamin and mineral supplements and diet), herbs, homeopathy and hydrotherapy. Massage, reflexology, and spinal manipulation can also be utilized effectively for restoration or maintenance of good health, although they are not covered extensively in this handbook.

This book is made up of two major sections. The first is **Nutrition**, which discusses the six classifications of nutrition as a major role in maintaining optimal health. The second part discusses specific **Ailments and Conditions**, including explanations, symptoms, causes, suggestions on what to do to achieve natural healing, including proposed supplementation* as well as suggestions as to what one can do to avoid the condition

This section of the book is not meant to provide quick relief for symptoms. When looking up a condition or ailment, it is important that you consider what the underlying causes are if you expect any relief from the symptoms. Elimination of the cause is often the best remedy to eliminate the symptoms. If you do not eliminate the cause and simply try to cover up the symptoms, you will encounter an unending cycle which can be more and more vicious with time.

For example, if you have dry skin, it is important to determine if a vitamin, mineral, or essential oil deficiency exists, or if over-exposure to the sun, or lack of humidity in the air, etc., is the cause in order for you to correct it. Creams and lotions are only a temporary solution which only cover up the symptom and will not solve the problem.

Another example is pain. Pain, such as a headache, can be due to any number of causes including allergies (food, inhalants, etc.), digestive problems (constipation, indigestion, toxicity, etc.), low blood sugar, stress, arthritis, over-indulgence in alcohol, high blood pressure, anemia, eye strain, and others. Pain killers may help your headache temporarily, but if the cause is not identified and eliminated, the headache is likely to return.

I would like to thank the numerous health authorities I have had the opportunity to work with in the last few years who have guided me and taught me a great deal about wholistic health and wellbeing. The following individuals have served as mentors to me and I am greatly indebted to each of them; Dr. Jeffrey Bland, Dr. Linus Pauling, Dr. Stephen Levine, Dr. Keith Sehnert, Dr. John Willard, Dr. Hal Huggins, Dr. Paul Eck, Dr. William McGarey, Dr. Oscar Rasmussen, Dr. Dean Call, Michael Tierra, Udo Erasmus, James South and finally, Dr. Arnold Susser, who is the author of the Foreword.

*This book is not intended to serve as medical advice. Its intention is solely informational and educational. Quantities shown for beneficial supplementation are not prescriptive. Some dosages are high and represent therapeutic test dosages. Individual needs and tolerances will vary according to body size, metabolism, age, diet and ailment. Please consult a medical or health professional should the need for one be warranted.

NOTE: Mega doses of certain nutrients such as vitamin are not recommended for prolonged periods unless one is under a doctor's supervision. Harmful levels may buildup in the body if high dosages are taken for prolonged periods.

Part I

Nutrition

Nutrition is the relationship between foods and the health of the body. Optimal nutrition is a diet that contains all essential nutrients which are supplied and utilized in a balanced amount to maintain health. Optimum dietary habits include two simple concepts: What you should eat and how much you should eat. Understanding the reasons behind these two concepts is a bit more complicated.

Knowledge of the nutrients and their functions in the body is needed for the understanding of good nutrition and a balanced diet. A balanced diet contains portions of each of the main nutrient classifications of food. The six basic classifications of nutrients are the carbohydrates, proteins, fats, vitamins, minerals, and water.

Each nutrient has its own special function and relationship to the body, but no nutrient acts independently of the other nutrients. All the nutrients must be present in the right quantities in order to maintain optimum health. Although everyone requires all these nutrients, individuals do not necessarily require the same amounts of these. Quantities vary according to individual needs.

The myth of the typical American diet is that it is normal, well-balanced, and contains sufficient amounts of all the nutrients we need.

The truth is it is not.

A balanced diet is often discussed in books, but many of us never actually see it in front of us. In spite of all the excuses we might have for not getting proper nutrients such as soil depletion, food processing and cooking, it ultimately is our own responsibility to feed ourselves properly. Just because a piece of white bread has all the natural nutrients refined out of it does not mean we have to eat it. There are many other much more nutritional food choices we can make.

We have become a nation of convenience. We want what is fast and easy. We have a huge abundance of fast food restaurants, frozen foods, canned foods, boxed foods and junk foods to choose from to satisfy our hunger and cravings. Unfortunately, the refining, preservatives and additives that accompany them are preventing us from

3

satisfying our nutritional needs.

Nationwide surveys in North America have shown that the diets of more than 60 percent of the people tested are deficient in one or more of the essential nutrients. The surveys tested only 10 of the 45 known nutrients, and used as their standard for adequate nutrition the very low Recommended Daily Allowances (RDA). These are recognized as the minimal requirements for these nutrients and are inadequate to maintain optimum health.

The most common deficiencies found in these surveys were iron, calcium, zinc, chromium, iodine, magnesium, selenium, manganese, vitamins C, A, E, B-6, B-2, folic acid, and essential fatty acids.

Nutritional deficiencies result whenever inadequate amounts of essential nutrients are provided to tissues over a long period of time. Good nutrition is essential for normal organ development and functioning, for normal reproduction, growth, for optimal energy and efficiency, for resistance to infection and disease, and for the ability to repair bodily damage or injury.

Deficiency symptoms are not necessarily obvious. Conditions develop slowly over time and are not black and white. One does not need to have scurvy to have a vitamin C deficiency. One does not need to have osteoporosis to have a calcium deficiency. Symptoms can be as subtle as appetite loss, bad breath, soft or brittle fingernails, fatigue, or insomnia.

Malnutrition does not only occur in areas of poverty or under-developed countries. We, one of the most technically advanced and fast paced nations, do not seem to know how to feed ourselves properly so we can feel our best.

We are not indestructible. One does not expect to feed an automobile diesel fuel while it requires unleaded and expect it to run optimally. Almost certainly it will end up at the service station accompanied by a hefty bill. Although a bit more complicated, humans fed improperly over time may end up at the hospital also accompanied by a hefty bill.

We are not exactly healthy as a population. We suffer

from colds, allergies, excessive weight, diabetes, hypoglycemia, anemia, arthritis, mental problems, heart disease, cancer and many other conditions that leave us unsatisfied with our health and feeling rotten. We too often do not even consider our own eating habits as the possible cause.

"Anyone who has in the past eaten sugar, white flour, or canned food has some deficiency disease..."

Dr. Daniel T. Quigley, author of "The National Malnutrition".

KNOWING YOUR A, B, Cs: VITAMINS

Vitamins are organic compounds which are indispensible to body functions. Vitamins are used within the body's various structures as building blocks and are necessary for various biochemical functions. Most vitamins must be ingested although some may be synthesized within the body.

In order to have optimum health, we must obtain an adequate quantity of each of the vitamins. The amount needed varies from person to person and the amounts of specific vitamins needed is based on a number of criteria. The Foods and Nutrition Board of the National Research Council have established Recommended Daily Allowances (RDA) for each of the vitamins, but many people disagree with this interpretation. For example, Nobel Prize winner Linus Pauling, believes that "the RDA for a vitamin is not the allowance that leads to the best of health for most people. It is, instead, only the estimated amount that for most people would prevent death or serious illness from overt vitamin deficiency."

In order to obtain optimum nutrition, many people use supplements in addition to eating a proper diet. Because nutrients in the soil are not as plentiful as they once were and many other factors, one cannot be certain the nutrient value of the foods eaten today.

Vitamins taken in excess of what can be utilized in the metabolic processes are not usually of any value and will either be excreted in the urine or stored in the body. Excessive consumption of some nutrients (particularly fat-soluble vitamins) may result in toxicity.

Vitamins are usually distinguished as being water-soluble or fat-soluble. The water-soluble vitamins are the B complex, C, and the bioflavonoids and are usually measured in milligrams. The fat-soluble vitamins are A, D, E, and K and are usually measured in International

Units (IU). An exception is beta carotene, a water-soluble form of vitamin A, which is expressed in IU also.

VITAMIN A:

An antioxidant essential for fat metabolism and to develop and maintain healthy skin, hair, nails, eyes (especially night vision), teeth, bones, gums, mucous linings, membranes, and various glands (especially the lungs). Vitamin A helps resist infection, and prevent premature aging and senility.

Natural sources: Whole milk, eggs, leafy green and yellow vegetables and fruit, and liver.

RDA: 5000 IU

BETA CAROTENE (PROVITAMIN A):

An excellent protective antioxidant. Beneficial for all functions of vitamin A. Beta carotene is water soluble and virtually non-toxic.

Natural sources: Beets, broccoli, carrots, cantaloupe, mustard, papaya, parsnips, pumpkin, spinach, sweet potatoes, tomatoes, watercress, and yellow string beans.

B-1 (THIAMINE):

Helps promote proper use of sugars and energy from food. Necessary for proper function of heart and nervous system. Thiamine is blood building, prevents fluid retention, prevents constipation and maintains muscle tone.

Natural sources: Whole grains and cereals, yeast, liver, pork, poultry, lean meat, eggs, and legumes.

RDA: 1.4 mg

B-2 (RIBOFLAVIN):

Aids in growth and reproduction, alleviates eye fatigue, aids in antibody and red blood cell formation, promotes healthy skin, hair, and nails, and aids in metabolism.

Natural sources: Milk, liver, cheese, fish, eggs, whole grains, brewer's yeast, almonds, and sunflower seeds.

RDA: 1.6 mg

8

B-3 (NIACIN):

Vital for use of carbohydrates, fats, and proteins, needed for formation of hormones, aids circulation (dilates blood vessels), controls cholesterol levels, and tones nervous system.

Natural sources: Liver, lean meat, poultry (white meat), fish, eggs, peanuts, avocados, dates, figs, prunes, green vegetables, whole wheat products, brewer's yeast, wheat germ, and rice bran.

RDA: 20 mg

B-5 (PANTOTHENIC ACID):

Formation of proteins and nucleic acids, helps maintain functions of the intestinal tract, prevents certain forms of anemia, aids in wound healing, antibody formation, growth stimulation and vitamin utilization.

Natural sources: Leafy green vegetables, beans, peas, nuts, liver, egg yolk, royal jelly, brewer's yeast, wheat germ, and wheat bran.

RDA: 10 mg

B-6: (PYRIDOXINE):

Facilitates the body's use of carbohydrates, proteins, and fats, needed for production of hydrochloric acid, alleviates nausea, needed for formation of antibodies.

Natural sources: Brewer's yeast, bananas, avocados, wheat germ, leafy green vegetables, whole grains and cereals, bananas, milk, eggs, blackstrap molasses, soybeans, walnuts, peanuts, and pecans.

RDA: 4 mcg

B-9 (FOLIC ACID):

Helps build red blood cells. Aids in body growth and reproduction, division of body cells, hydrochloric acid production, and protein metabolism.

Natural sources: Brewer's yeast, leafy deep green vegetables, wheat germ, mushrooms, nuts, liver, broccoli, asparagus, lima beans, and lettuce.

RDA: 4 mcg

B-12 (COBALAMIN):

Needed for formation of blood cells, increases energy and memory, needed for metabolism (fats, carbohydrates, and protein) and promotes growth.

Natural sources: Kelp, bananas, peanuts, concord grapes, sunflower seeds, brewer's yeast, wheat germ, bee pollen, liver, beef, eggs, pork, milk, and cheese.

RDA: 6 mcg

B-13 (OROTIC ACID):

Essential for synthesis of nucleic acid and regenerative processes in cells.

Natural sources: Root vegetables, whey, the liquid portion of soured or curdled milk.

RDA not established

B-15 (CALCIUM PANGAMATE):

Aids in recovery from fatigue, cell oxidation and respiration, metabolism (carbohydrate, fat, sugar) glandular and nervous system stimulation.

Natural sources: Whole grains, whole brown rice, pumpkin seeds, sesame seeds, nuts, and brewer's yeast.

RDA not established

B-17 (LAETRILE):

Thought to have cancer controlling and preventative properties.

Natural sources: Whole seeds (apricot, peach, and plum pits) mung beans, lima beans, garbanzo beans, blackberries, blueberries, cranberries, raspberries, millet and flaxseed.

RDA not established

BIOTIN:

Is an antiseptic, and is needed for cell growth and fatty acid production, hair growth, metabolism, and vitamin B utilization.

Natural sources: Brewer's yeast, fruits, nuts, soybeans, unpolished rice, beef, liver, egg yolk, and milk.

RDA: 3 mcg

CHOLINE:

Controls cholesterol buildup, lecithin formation, liver and gall bladder regulation, lowers blood pressure, nerve transmission.

Natural sources: Granular or liquid lecithin, brewer's yeast, wheat germ, egg yolk, liver, and green leafy vegetables.

RDA not established

INOSITOL:

Provides a calming effect, helps reduce cholesterol and slows artery hardening, prevents eczema, needed for hair growth and metabolism.

Natural sources: Liver, brewer's yeast, cabbage, citrus fruits, cantaloupe, raisins, wheat germ, whole grains, peanuts, lecithin, milk, and unrefined molasses.

RDA not established

PABA (PARA-AMINOBENZOIC ACID):

Aids in blood cell formation, reproductive disorders, restoration of graying hair, maintenance of intestinal bacteria and has important sun-screen properties.

Natural sources: Liver, kidney, molasses, brewer's yeast, rice bran, whole grains, wheat germ, vegetables, peas, beans, peanuts, and egg yolk.

RDA not established

C (ASCORBIC ACID):

Accelerates healing, needed for bone and teeth formation, collagen production, prevention of common cold, digestion, red blood cell formation, shock and infection resistance, thought to have cancer protection agents.

Natural sources: Rose hips, citrus fruits, black currants, berries, broccoli, cabbage, cauliflower, persimmons, guavas, sweet potatoes, and green bell peppers.

RDA: 60 mg

11

D (ERGOSTEROL, CALCIFEROL, VIOSTEROL):

Needed for strong teeth and bones, heart action, nervous system maintenance, normal blood clotting and skin respiration. Helps utilize vitamin A, calcium and phosphorus properly. Vitamin D can be acquired through sunlight. Ultraviolet rays act on the oils of the skin to produce the vitamin, which is then absorbed into the body.

Natural sources: Milk, fish liver oil, egg yolk, tuna, salmon, sardines, herring, sprouted seeds, mushrooms, and sunflower seeds.

RDA: 400 IU

E (TOCOPHEROL):

Anti-coagulant, antioxidant, alleviates fatigue, dilates blood vessels, blood cholesterol reduction, improves circulation, capillary formation and functioning of red blood cells, muscle, and other tissues, protects essential fatty acids.

Natural sources: Vegetable oils, whole grain cereals, wheat germ, lettuce, brussels sprouts, leafy greens, soybeans, and eggs.

RDA: 10 mg (12-15 IU)

F (LINOLEIC AND LINOLENIC ESSENTIAL FATTY ACIDS):

Needed for blood coagulation, for normal blood pressure, to control cholesterol, to combat heart disease, for healthy hair, skin and for normal glandular activity.

Natural Sources: Vegetable oils, flax, wheat germ, almonds, avocados, peanuts, sunflower seeds, walnuts, soybeans, and safflower.

RDA not established

K (MENADIONE):

Required for normal blood clotting, activates energy producing tissues and is important for the liver.

Natural sources: Kelp, alfalfa, yogurt, egg yolk, safflower and soybean oil, fish liver oil, and leafy green vegetables.

RDA not established

Vitamins and Enzymes

Vitamins are components of our enzyme system, which energize and regulate our metabolism. Vitamins function with enzymes. Enzymes are made up of two parts: A protein molecule and a coenzyme. This coenzyme may be a vitamin, may contain a vitamin, or may be a molecule that has been manufactured from a vitamin.

Enzymes are substances charged with vital energy factors responsible for the oxidation process. They hold both biological and chemical properties. In the body, enzymes cause or speed up chemical reactions. Enzymes are required for every chemical reaction that occurs in the body. There are three types of enzymes: metabolic enzymes (which run our bodies), digestive enzymes (which digest our food), and food enzymes (which start food digestion).

Since good health depends on all of these metabolic enzymes doing an excellent job, it is necessary to be sure nothing interferes with the body's ability to make enough of them. A shortage could mean trouble. Hundreds of enzymes are necessary to carry on the work of the body-to repair damage and decay, and heal diseases.

Digestive Enzymes

The enzymes most familiar to many of us are the digestive enzymes. Their main responsibility is to digest the food we eat so we can benefit from it. Protease enzymes digest protein, amylase enzymes digest carbohydrates, and lipase enzymes digest fat.

Food enzymes help with digestion by doing some of the work so the body's digestive enzymes need not be totally responsible. Our main digestive organ, the pancreas, produces some of these digestive enzymes. However, food enzymes are necessary so the pancreas is not overburdened. The pancreas is crucial to the digestion of all kinds of food, providing all three types of digestive enzymes.

Digestion is the first step in the conversion of food to

13

energy. Everything the body needs for optimal health is taken from what we eat as it passes through the digestive tract. Except for water and salt, these foods must be converted into simple sugars, amino acids and free fatty acids to be used by the body. This is accomplished with the help of the various enzymes embedded in cells on the lining of the stomach and small intestine. Acids from inside the stomach also aid digestion.

After broken down into their essential nutrients, assorted food molecules are absorbed through the enzyme-embedded cells into the blood and lymph system. The nutrients are then made available to the tissues throughout the body. Without these enzymes the vitamins, minerals, and other nutrients in the foods we eat would have no value.

For optimal health, food enzymes are necessary. Food enzymes must come from uncooked foods such as fresh fruits and vegetables, raw sprouted grains, unpasteurized dairy products, and from enzyme supplements. When foods are cooked, the enzyme content is destroyed and the body must supply all the enzymes for digestion.

When we consume enzymes from raw foods or supplementation, the body does not have to use up its own supply. When food enzymes take over some of the work, according to the Law of Adaptive Secretion of Digestive Enzymes, the enzyme potential can allot less activity to digestive enzymes, and have more to give to the hundreds of metabolic enzymes that run the entire body.

When an excessive amount of digestive enzymes must be produced, the body, especially the pancreas, is stressed and the enzyme potential may be unable to produce an adequate quantity of metabolic enzymes to repair body organs and fight disease.

Supplemental enzymes can help prevent this and are usually available in two types: pancreatic and all-vegetative. Vegetative enzymes work in the stomach similar to food enzymes. Pancreatic enzymes work in the alkaline environment of the small intestine. They are usually available in an enteric coated form which protects them from the acidity of the stomach.

MINERALS

Minerals are another group of essential nutrients needed for our physical and mental health. In the body they form part of tissue structures and are components of important organic molecules such as enzymes and hormones which regulate all processes such as the immune system, growth and energy in the body. Each of these enzymes and hormones depend on minerals and trace minerals to function. Minerals help to regulate the flow of fluids and maintain water and acid-base balance in the body. Minerals have the power to rejuvenate energy, to overcome fatigue, and to improve thinking and memory. They facilitate nerve impulse transmission and muscle contraction and help strengthen the nervous and skeletal system. In addition, minerals are needed to grow new hair, to normalize the heart beat, and much more.

The body functions best when all the needed nutrients, including minerals, are present in their proper proportions. But if there is a shortage of just one mineral, the system will weaken and begin to lose efficiency. In fact, in the absence of minerals, vitamins have no function. Lacking vitamins, the body can still make use of minerals, but lacking minerals, vitamins are useless. With the balance of the body off, functions of the body cannot operate optimally and eventually disease will set in.

Deficiencies

For a number of reasons, individuals often do not get all they need of some minerals in their diet. Food plants are grown in soil deficient in important minerals because synthetic and super-phosphate fertilizers, pesticides, herbicides, growth regulators, and livestock feed additives destroy microbial soil life needed to make the soil nutrients available to the plant. In addition, many of the minerals are in the form of water soluble salts, and unfortunately rains and heavy irrigation over the years

15

can wash away these salts, causing depleted soil conditions.

Variable amounts of minerals are lost because of cooking and processing. Food preservation methods such as blanching, freezing, and smoking cause up to a 30 percent nutrient loss and canning and sun-drying can cause up to a 50 percent loss of nutrients. Chemical additives may have protective, destructive or no effects on the nutrients in the foods.

Losses due to cooking varies with the method used, amount of water used, cooking time and several other variables. Boiling (cooking foods in water at a temperature of 212 degrees F.) can cause significant nutrient losses. Minerals are lost when large amounts of water encourage leaching. Best retention of vitamins and minerals is achieved when cooking with as little water as possible and for as little time as possible. Steaming causes fewer nutrient losses than boiling does. Mineral losses from steaming average approximately half of what they would have been for boiling. Microwave cooking is not necessarily better than conventional cooking methods. Roasting or stewing can lead to greater loss of some nutrients than boiling does.

Bioavailability

Many individuals also have trouble assimilating and utilizing minerals even from highly assimilable food sources. Although healthy people generally absorb more than 90 percent of the protein, carbohydrate, and fat in their diets, they do not generally absorb minerals as efficiently. In fact, in controlled studies, adults have been found to absorb an average of only about five percent of the manganese, 10 percent of the iron, 10-20 percent of the zinc, and 30-40 percent of the magnesium and calcium from their diets.

Foods and medications that individuals consume can cause large variations in the bioavailability of minerals in their diets. For example, healthy adults have been found to absorb anywhere from one percent to over 35 percent of their dietary iron intake, depending on the composition of their diets and the same absorption applies for zinc. Bioavailability of minerals can also be influenced by several other factors.

For example, a high fiber diet can interfere with the uptake of many minerals since it contains substances which combine with minerals to form insoluble compounds. In addition, fiber helps food move through the digestive tract faster allowing less time for absorption of minerals.

Because diet alone may not provide all the needed minerals one needs, many nutritionists suggest combining a diet high in unprocessed and unrefined foods with adequate supplementation of the necessary minerals which anticipate the problems of assimilation.

Major and Minor

Major minerals are those found in larger amounts in the body such as calcium and magnesium and trace minerals are found in very minute amounts such as chromium and selenium. They are all necessary for normal functioning of the body. The following is a brief explanation of a few of the major and trace minerals, showing their importance to our health and the prevention of disease:

ALUMINUM is found in all tissues and is believed to be required in trace amounts in some enzyme functions. It can be dangerous, however, if consumed in excessive amounts. Most of the harmful effects of aluminum result from the destruction of vitamins. Cooking in aluminum utensils and using food stored in aluminum containers should be avoided.

Aluminum is found in tap water, baking powder, table salt (added to prevent caking), some stomach antacids, and some processed cheeses.

CALCIUM is the most abundant mineral in the body with about 99 percent deposited in the bones and teeth.

Soft tissues and blood contain the remaining. The main function of calcium is to act in cooperation with phosphorus to build and maintain bones and teeth. It is also essential for healthy blood, helps regulate the heartbeat, is needed for nerve and muscle stimulation and for blood clotting processes. Calcium normally needs strong stomach acid secretions and usually only about 20 percent is absorbed.

Calcium is found in significant amounts in milk and dairy products, but also is found in smaller amounts in fish, seaweed, blackstrap molasses, nuts and seeds, black beans, soybeans, tofu, and vegetable greens.

CHLORINE is an essential mineral occurring in the body mainly in compound form with sodium or potassium. Chlorine helps regulate the correct balance of acid and alkali in the blood and maintains pressure that causes fluid to pass through cell membranes. It also stimulates the production of hydrochloric acid in the stomach which is needed for digestion of protein and high fiber foods.

Chlorine is found largely in table salt, but also in kelp, dulse, rye flour, ripe olives, and sea greens.

CHROMIUM is needed to escort glucose through cell walls. Insulin requires the cooperation of infinite amounts of chromium as a catalyst. Many documented cases of diabetes have resulted from a diet of chromium-poor processed foods and could have been prevented by the use of chromium-rich foods such as brewer's yeast, beef liver, chicken, whole grains or supplements.

COBALT is considered an essential mineral and is an integral part of vitamin B-12 (cobalamin). Cobalt activates a number of enzymes in the body, is necessary for normal functioning and maintenance of red blood cells as well as other body cells.

Cobalt is found readily in meats, oysters, clams, and milk.

18

COPPER is found in all body tissues. It assists in the formation of hemoglobin and red blood cells by facilitating iron absorption. Copper is present in enzymes that break up or build up body tissues. It also is involved in healing and protein metabolism.

Copper is found in liver, whole grain products, almonds, green leafy vegetables, dried legumes, and most seafood.

FLUORINE is an essential nutrient that is present in very minute amounts in almost all human tissues. It is found primarily in the bones and teeth. There are two types of fluorine: sodium fluoride which is added to our drinking water and is not the same as calcium fluoride, which is found in nature. Excessive fluorine in the body is harmful because it can destroy some enzymes which are vital to many body processes such as the metabolism of vitamins.

Fluorinated water (sodium fluoride) is the most common source of fluorine, although this form may be toxic. Other sources of fluorine are seafood, cheese, meat, and tea.

IODINE is converted in the body into iodide. The body contains about 50 milligrams of this element. About 10-15 milligrams are located in the thyroid gland where it is oxidized and converted to the hormone thyroxine. This hormone regulates the body's energy production, rate of metabolism, carbohydrate absorption, conversion of carotene to vitamin A and it regulates pulse and heart beat.

Iodine is found in seafood and sea greens, mushrooms and irish moss.

IRON is a very temperamental mineral requiring adequate systemic amounts of vitamin C, calcium, copper, cobalt, vitamin E, vitamin F, and 19 different amino acids in order to be absorbed. It is concentrated in the blood and is essential for the formation of hemoglobin and myoglobin which transport oxygen throughout the body.

Iron is found in liver, oysters, heart, lean meat, leafy green vegetables, whole grains, dried fruits, legumes, and molasses.

MAGNESIUM is an essential mineral element found inside all cells where it is involved in many metabolic processes. The functions of magnesium include enzyme reactions, energy release (ATP), neuromuscular contraction, calcium absorption, protein synthesis and body temperature regulation. It also helps utilization of vitamin C, vitamin E, and the B Complex. Because magnesium is very alkaline, it helps regulate the acid-alkaline balance of the body.

Magnesium is found in fresh green vegetables, raw, unmilled wheat germ, soybeans, milk, whole grains, seafood, figs, corn, apples, and almonds.

MANGANESE is vital to the development of bones, ligaments, nerves and also is important to proper digestion. It is also important in sex hormone and milk production and functions as a catalyst and enzyme activator. Recent studies show a manganese deficiency contributes to excess blood sugar.

Manganese is found in whole-grain cereals, egg yolks, nuts, seeds, and green vegetables. **NOTE:** A great deal of manganese is lost in the processing and milling of foods.

PHOSPHORUS is the second most abundant mineral in the body. It functions with vitamin D and calcium and is found in every cell in the body. It is essential for energy production, muscle contraction, digestion and the pH balance of the blood.

Food sources of phosphorus include meat, fish, poultry, eggs, whole grains, and seeds.

POTASSIUM is the third most abundant mineral in the body and constitutes approximately five percent of total mineral content. Potassium is an essential mineral found in intracellular fluid and is very important to

20

electrical, nerve, muscle and heart functions. Potassium is water soluble and works with sodium to normalize heartbeat. Potassium, sodium and chloride help regulate the water balance in the body. Rapid water loss can deplete potassium from the body with serious consequences.

Potassium is contained in all vegetables, oranges, whole grains, sunflower seeds and mint leaves.

SELENIUM is a trace mineral that is often known to be interdependent with vitamin E. In some instances a low level of one nutrient can be partly compensated for by the presence of the other. Selenium is a component of an important enzyme that helps prevent damage to cell structure. Some studies have shown that selenium has a protective effect.

Food sources of selenium include brewer's yeast, organ and muscle meats, fish and shellfish, grains, cereals, and dairy products.

SILICON is present in the skeletal structures and connective tissues in the body such as cartilage, tendons and blood vessels. Silicon, phosphorus and calcium combine to make strong bones and could be an important factor in osteoporosis and atherosclerosis.

The best sources of silicon are hard drinking water and plant fiber.

SODIUM functions with potassium in keeping blood minerals soluble. Together with chloride they balance the electrolyte cell function and equalize the acid-alkali factor in the blood.

Sodium is found ia almost all foods, especially salt, kelp, seafood, poultry and meat.

SULFUR is a non-metallic element present in every cell. It is prevalent in keratin, a tough protein which is important for the skin, hair and nails. It is necessary for collagen synthesis. The hormone insulin contains a large amount of sulfur and is essential in the regulation of carbohydrate metabolism.

Sulfur is not readily found in the diet largely due to soil depletion. The best source of sulfur is eggs, but it is found in small amounts in meat, fish, cheese, and milk.

VANADIUM is present in most body tissues and is considered essential to human health. Bones, cartilage, and teeth require vanadium for proper development.

Vanadium is commonly lost in food processing, but best sources include fats, oils, whole grains, seafood and meats.

ZINC is essential for proper development of reproductive organs and health of the prostrate gland. It is also necessary for proper B vitamin utilization, digestion, healing and the synthesis of nucleic acid. Extensive zinc depletion can have serious effects on the immune system especially when fighting against degenerative diseases. A zinc deficiency is also a factor in stress, fatigue, loss or taste or smell and decreased alertness. At least 25 enzymes are dependent on zinc.

Zinc is found in protein foods such as meat, unprocessed whole-grain products, brewer's yeast, wheat bran, wheat germ, and pumpkin seeds.

Mineral Balancing

Obtaining enough minerals through the diet is only half of the battle. The other half is maintaining balanced levels among each of the minerals. Dr. Paul Eck, scientist and mineral researcher, is probably recognized as one of the foremost authorities in the world on the role of minerals in human health. One of the main points he stresses is that mineral imbalance is the underlying cause of most of our health troubles.

For example, according to Dr. Eck, the four main minerals in the body regulate two areas of critical importance in the body, the thyroid and adrenal glands: Calcium, magnesium, sodium, and potassium. If these four minerals are at normal levels, and everything else is in balance, these glands can function optimally.

Imbalances will cause either over-activity which can result in stress or under activity which results in low energy levels and insufficiency. For example, calcium and potassium are the two major minerals involved in the activity of the thyroid gland. If the ratio between them and the minerals levels are normal, the thyroid functions at maximum energy levels. Calcium acts to slow down the activity of the thyroid and potassium speeds it up. If the level of calcium is too high the energy level of the thyroid will be slowed down. If the level of potassium is too high the thyroid will be overactive and will eventually wear out completely because of too much stress.

Magnesium and sodium are the minerals associated with the adrenal gland. Too much magnesium in relation to sodium will slow down the adrenal gland. Too much sodium in relation to magnesium will speed up the adrenal glands. According to Eck, one can tell how healthy a person's adrenal glands are by evaluating his sodium and magnesium levels. The same goes for all other glands in the body.

Also, if just one mineral level is too high or too low, it affects all other minerals in the body because no mineral works alone. For example, commonly individuals take an iron supplement because they are tired. This is what can happen: Iron causes sodium levels to rise as a result of stimulating the adrenal glands. Magnesium levels will go down because sodium lowers magnesium. Calcium will go down because magnesium and calcium strive to be at the same level. Calcium and potassium move in opposite directions, so when calcium goes down, potassium goes up. It doesn't end here, since as many as 21 minerals can be affected by alternating just one. Again, no mineral works alone.

CARBOHYDRATES

Carbohydrates are the chief source of energy for all body functions and muscle uses. They are also needed for the digestion and assimilation of other foods. Carbohydrates provide immediate available calories for energy by producing heat when carbon in the system unites with oxygen in the bloodstream. Carbohydrates also help regulate protein and fat metabolism; fats require carbohydrates for their breakdown within the liver.

The principal carbohydrates present in foods are divided into groups. The simple carbohydrates are the mono-saccharides, disaccharides, trisaccharides, and oligosaccharides. The complex carbohydrates are the polysaccharides.

Monosaccharides are considered "simple sugars." They contain a one monomeric unit sugar molecule such as glucose, fructose, galactose, dextrose and about 200 others. Glucose is the most abundant in nature.

Disaccharides contain two monosaccharide molecules combined chemically. Examples are lactose (found in milk), galactose (found in sugar beets), maltose (found in beer), and sucrose (table sugar).

Trisaccharides contain three monomeric sugar molecules. An example is raffinose, which is abundant in sugar beets.

An oligosaccharide contains up to 10 sugar molecules. Polysaccharides contain many hundreds or thousands of molecules and may contain more than one type of monomer.

Amylose, amylopectin, glycogen (animal starch), and cellulose are examples of polysaccharides.

Most starches are considered complex carbohydrates when unrefined. Starches are sugar molecules bonded together. Enzymes in the body break down the bonds between the sugar molecules and turn starches into sugars. One starch molecule contains 4,000-30,000 glucose molecules chemically combined. Cellulose has about 3,000 glucose molecules.

In general, the more complex the carbohydrate is the longer it takes to digest. Some polysaccharides are not digested at all and are an excellent source of fiber. Examples are cellulose which is found in celery, inulin which is found in Jerusalem artichokes, and agar which is found in some types of seaweed.

All other carbohydrates are converted in the body to a simple sugar such as glucose or fructose. Some of the blood sugar is used as fuel by tissues in the brain, nervous system, and muscles. A small portion of the glucose is converted to glycogen and stored by the liver and muscles. The excess is converted to fat and stored throughout the body. When fat reserves are needed for energy and converted to glucose to be used as body fuel, weight loss results.

Many nutritionists assume that starch molecules, which require a two step digestion process because they contain long chains of glucose (or other types of sugar) molecules, would be digested and reach the blood stream much more slowly than a simple sugar like glucose or even a slightly more complex sugar like sucrose. But, laboratory tests show this is not the case. Starches begin the digestion process in the mouth with saliva. Even so, starches are considered a complex carbohydrate, provided they are unrefined, because of their nutritional value.

Refined starches include white flour, white rice, pasta, enriched flours (both white and dark), corn starch, tapioca, and most breakfast cereals found on supermarket shelves, as well as all the products made with these ingredients.

Unrefined starches are not usually as detrimental to blood sugar levels because they are more complex and are rich in vitamin and mineral co-factors needed by the body. These are starchy vegetables and fruits, yams, potatoes, corn, figs, bananas, and the many varieties of grains. The main source of carbohydrates should be complex carbohydrates like fruits, vegetables, beans, nuts, seeds, and whole grain breads, cereals and other complex unrefined starches.

Complex carbohydrates take much longer to metabolize in comparison to simple carbohydrates. In general, the more unrefined the carbohydrate, the longer the time required (with the exception of starches). These carbohydrates release a slow, constant stream of glucose into the blood stream and therefore, produce less impact upon the blood sugar levels.

Complex-Unrefined

All vegetables
All whole grains
All whole cereals
Nuts
Seeds
Legumes
Greens

Complex-Refined

Flour
Cornstarch
White rice
Potato starch
Bread, crackers
Pasta

Simple-Unrefined

All fruit
Milk
Yogurt
Buttermilk
Raw honey
Sugar cane
Molasses

Simple-Refined

Sugar
Honey
Corn syrup (dextrose)
Fructose
Lactose
Glucose
Maltose
Maple sugar
Sorbitol

How Much?

Traditionally, carbohydrates are a part of every meal in the form of a starch serving such as potatoes or rice, a vegetable serving and a fruit serving. These guidelines are not bad for a start but there is more to it than just that.

Recommendations for carbohydrate intake are usually up to 60 percent of total daily calorie intake (which should be almost entirely complex). Carbohydrates yield approximately 4 calories per gram. For example, according to this recommendation:

A man who consumes 2600 calories daily would require approximately 1500 calories or 370 grams of carbohydrates.

A woman who consumes 2000 calories daily would require approximately 1200 calories or 300 grams of carbohydrates.

The following examples of foods show the possible suppliers of carbohydrates.

* One cup 40% bran flakes cereal (without milk or sweetener)
    152 calories
    37.3 grams of carbohydrates (mostly complex)

* One slice whole wheat bread
    56 calories
    11 grams carbohydrates (mostly complex)

* One cake doughnut
    125 calories
    16.4 grams carbohydrates (simple, refined)

* One cup chocolate pudding
    385 calories
    66.8 grams carbohydrates (simple, refined)

* One-half cup brown rice
    300 calories
    75 grams carbohydrates (mostly complex, unrefined)

* One apple
    80 calories
    21 grams carbohydrates (simple, unrefined)

* One cup fresh grape juice
155 calories
37.8 grams carbohydrates (simple, unrefined)

* One-half cup cashews
350 calories
20 grams carbohydrates (unrefined, complex)

* One cup green peas
122 calories
21 grams carbohydrates (unrefined, complex)

* One large baked potato
145 calories
26 grams carbohydrates (unrefined, complex)

A lack of dietary carbohydrates can result in fatigue, depression, breakdown of body protein and mineral imbalance.

Excess carbohydrates will be converted to simple sugars and then stored in the liver as glycogen which can eventually change into fatty acids which are stored in the tissues or organs.

Foods rich in carbohydrates are described in the following:

Whole grains

Grains are often referred to as cereals. They are the seeds of various grasses such as wheat, rye, oats, rice and barley. The entire grain is edible and full of nutrients. Most whole grains are especially rich in B vitamins, vitamin E, protein, complex carbohydrates, unsaturated fatty acids, and minerals (especially iron). In processing to make flour, bread, breakfast cereals, and macaroni, most of these nutrients are lost.

Whole brown rice is high in B vitamins, and also contains calcium, phosphorus, and iron. Wild rice contains twice as much protein, four times as much phosphorus, eight times as much thiamine, and 20 times as much riboflavin as white rice. White rice (refined, dehulled polished rice) contains no significant amount of B vitamins.

Vegetables

Vegetables are primarily composed of carbohydrates and water and contain very little protein. Vegetables also provide vitamins, minerals and fiber to the diet. In general, light green vegetables provide vitamins, minerals, and a large amount of cellulose, necessary for bulk.

Yellow and dark green vegetables are excellent sources of vitamin A. Vegetable leaves are usually rich in calcium, iron, magnesium, potassium, vitamin C and many of the B vitamins. The greener the leaf, the richer it will be in nutrients. Potatoes contain some protein and are excellent sources of vitamin A, vitamin C, niacin, thiamine, and riboflavin, iron, calcium and potassium.

It is best to rely upon fresh and raw vegetables if at all possible. Fresh vegetables generally contain more vitamins and minerals than processed products. Quick-freezing is not as damaging to nutrient content. Properly canned vegetables can contain about the same nutrient value as home-cooked fresh vegetables. Dried vegetables have a significant loss of nutrients.

Before fresh vegetables are eaten or cooked, they should be thoroughly washed to remove chemical sprays and dirt. Vegetable skins should be left on or pared as thinly as possible to retain mineral and vitamin content. Cooking time should be kept to the absolute minimum. Steaming will retain more nutrient content in comparison to boiling. At least half of the minerals will be retained by steaming that would have been lost by boiling.

Baked vegetables will also have a higher concentration of nutrients than boiled vegetables. However, vegetables baked in juices (roasting) will lose more of some vitamins than if boiled. Cooking can breakup complex carbohydrates and change them into simple carbohydrates. For example, cooked potatoes and white rice are high in simple carbohydrates.

30

To obtain the maximum benefits of vegetables, eat them fresh and raw. This way one can be assured they have not lost nutrients and are complex.

Many individuals are low in mineral levels, largely and simply because they do not eat enough vegetables. Vegetables also provide essential fatty acids which many people are deficient in, sterols which reduce cholesterol, and fiber which is a necessity for regular elimination. Cooking and processing also destroy fiber and essential fatty acids.

There are a wide variety of vegetables that can be enjoyed by adding them to the diet. Some of these are:

Alfalfa sprouts
Artichokes
  (Jerusalem & Globe)
Asparagus
Black-eyed peas
Beets
Beet greens
Broccoli
Brussels sprouts
Cabbage
Carrots
Cauliflower
Celery
Chard
Chives
Collards
Corn
Cucumbers
Eggplant
Endive
Garlic
Green beans
Kale
Kohlrabi
Leeks

Lettuce (Boston, Romaine, & Iceberg)
Mushrooms
Mung bean sprouts
Okra
Onions
Parsley
Parsnips
Peas (Split and Green)
Peppers
  (Red, Green & Yellow)
Pimentos
Potatoes
Pumpkin
Radishes
*Rutabaga
Spinach
Squash
  (Summer and Winter)
Sweet potatoes
Turnips
Turnip greens
Water chestnuts
Watercress
Yams

* contains at least 5 percent glucose

31

Fruit

Fresh fruits are good sources of vitamins (especially A and C), minerals, enzymes, carbohydrates in the form of cellulose and natural sugars, and water. Fresh, raw fruits make satisfying and nutritious substitutions for refined carbohydrate foods like cake, cookies, sweet rolls, and candy, which contain few nutrients. Yellow fruits, such as apricots, cantaloupe, and persimmons, are good sources of beta carotene, which converts to vitamin A in the body. Acerola cherries, rose hips, cantaloupe, strawberries, tomatoes and the citrus fruits (oranges, grapefruit, lemons, and tangerines) are good sources of vitamin C.

Many fruits like bananas and apples contain significant amounts of fiber to aid in digestion. Bananas are especially high in potassium and magnesium, minerals individuals are commonly deficient in.

Fruits taste sweet and are a far superior food choice to sugary desserts and candy because of the nutrients they contain. Most fruits contain a mixture of fructose (also called levulose), and glucose. Glucose sugar requires insulin to be used in the body but fructose does not. Because of this, fructose and many fruits can be tolerated in moderation even by sugar sensitive individuals like hypoglycemics.

Fruits that are over-ripe are higher in sugar. Dried fruits are also high in sugar. Raisins are 70 percent sugar and plums contain 30 percent glucose plus 15 percent fructose. Some individuals such as hypoglycemics may with to avoid fruits that are over-ripe or dried due to their high sugar content.

Green fruits often contain enzyme inhibitors and should be allowed to ripen at room temperature and then stored in a cool, dark place such as the refrigerator.

NOTE: Avocados are a useful dietary choice for hypoglycemic individuals. Avocados contain a seven-carbon sugar which actually depresses insulin production, making this fruit an excellent choice (although possibly unwise for diabetics). Avocados also contain a significant amount of essential fatty acids.

Fruits should always be washed prior to eating to remove any existing chemical residue. Skins should be eaten to obtain maximum nutrient benefits.

Raw fruits contain the maximum nutrient, enzyme and fiber content. Cooking, canning, drying, and freezing decreases the nutrient value of the fruits.

There are a wide variety of fruits that are nutritious and can healthfully satisfy a sweet tooth. A few are listed below:

Apple
Apricot
Avocado
*Banana
Blackberries
Black currants
Blueberries
Boysenberries
*Cherries
Crabapple
Cranberries
Elderberries
*Figs
Gooseberries
Grapefruit
Grapes, Concord
*Grapes, white
Guava
Kiwi fruit
Kumquat
Lemon
Lime
Loganberries

*Loquat
Mango
Melon (Cantaloupe,
    Casaba & Honeydew)
Mulberries
Nectarine
Orange
Papaya
Passion Fruit
Peach
Pear
Persimmon
Pineapple, ripened on
    plant
*Pineapple, picked green
Pomegranate
Prunes, uncooked
Raspberries
Rhubarb
Strawberries
Tangerine
Watermelon

*contains at least 5 percent glucose

33

FATS

Fats are the most concentrated source of energy in the diet. When oxidized, fats furnish more than twice the number of calories per gram furnished by carbohydrates or proteins.

Fats serve many vital functions in the body in addition to supplying the body with energy. Fatty acids are the major structural component of the membranes which surround cells, and within each cell, of the membranes which surround subcellular organelles. Therefore, fatty acids have important functions in the maintenance and building of healthy cells.

Fats also act as carriers of fat-soluble vitamins A, D, E, and K. Fats are also important in the conversion of beta carotene to vitamin A. Fat deposits surround, protect, and hold in place organs, such as the liver, kidneys, and heart. A layer of fat also insulates and protects the body from environmental temperature changes and preserves body heat.

Fatty acids are the major building blocks of the fats within our bodies and foods which are important sources of energy for the body.

Saturated vs. Unsaturated

Saturated fatty acids are solid at room temperature and are usually found in animal products. Saturated vegetable fats are found in many solid and "hydrogenated" shortenings, such as coconut oil and cocoa butter. **NOTE:** These are sometimes advertised as "cholesterol free," which is true, but may be misleading because these fats are unhealthy and should be avoided.

Saturated fats are metabolized more slowly by the body when compared to unsaturated fats. Saturated fats should be avoided in the diet because they tend to raise serum cholesterol levels in the body. Elevated cholesterol levels in the blood have been associated with an increased risk for the development of coronary heart disease.

35

Because many saturated fatty acids occur naturally in animal products and cannot be eliminated completely, try to cut down whenever possible, for example, remove skin on poultry before cooking.

Foods high in saturated fat include: (Estimated percentages given are of total fat contained.)

Coconut oil *(89% saturated)* and coconut butter
Palm and palm kernel oil *(46% saturated)*
Cottonseed oil *(23% saturated)*
Butter *(60% saturated)*
Hard cheese, i.e. chedder *(63% saturated)*
Cream cheese *(64% saturated)*
Beef fat *(50% saturated)*
Pork, all cuts, i.e. Bacon *(37% saturated)*
Lamb chops *(54% saturated)*

Unsaturated fatty acids usually are liquid at room temperature and many are from vegetable sources like safflower, soy, and corn. Other sources of unsaturated fatty acids are wheat germ, seeds, and cod liver oil. Whole grains and green leafy vegetables are very low in fat but the fat they do contain is unsaturated. Many animal products are high in monounsaturated fats, but are not recommended because of their contents of cholesterol and saturated fat.

Unsaturated fatty acids are important for respiration of vital organs and make it easier for oxygen to be transported by the bloodstream to all cells, tissues and organs. Unsaturated fatty acids also regulate blood flow and help break up cholesterol deposits on arterial walls. They are essential for normal glandular activity, especially for that of the adrenals and thyroid. They nourish and maintain the health of the skin, mucous membranes and nerves and have many, many more important functions.

Monounsaturated fats in the diet seem to have no effect on total serum cholesterol levels and do not lower the good-cholesterol-high density lipoprotein (HDL). Polyunsaturated fats in the diet tend to lower serum cholesterol levels.

Foods high in monunsaturated fats include: (Estimated percentages given are of total fat contained.)

Olives and olive oil *(77% monounsaturated)*
Canola (rapeseed) oil *(62% monounsaturated)*
Vegetable shortening *(50% monunsaturated)*
Margarine *(49% monounsaturated)*
Peanuts and peanut oil *(49% monunsaturated)*
Sunflower seed oil *(20% monounsaturated)*
Avocados *(75% monunsaturated)*
Most nuts (except coconut and walnuts)

Foods high in polyunsaturated fats include:

Safflower oil
Sunflower seeds and oil
Corn oil
Soybean oil
Walnuts and peanuts

Cholesterol

Cholesterol is a lipid or fat-related substance necessary for good health. We are provided the small amount of cholesterol we need in two ways. Cholesterol is naturally synthesized in the body by the liver and is also found in all animal products such as meat, seafood, dairy products and eggs. Egg yolks and organ meats are very high in cholesterol. Although low in total fat, shrimp, lobster and sardines are fairly high in cholesterol. Foods of plant origin such as fruits, vegetables, grains, cereals, nuts and seeds contain no cholesterol .

While deficiencies of cholesterol in the body are unlikely to occur, excessive amount of cholesterol commonly accumulate throughout the body if fats are eaten excessively.

Lecithin (found in egg yolks, liver, nuts, whole wheat, unrefined vegetable oils, soybeans and corn), inositol, and the essential fatty acids are important dietary factors which help break up and transport cholesterol in the body. Also important are fiber, Vitamins A, D, and C .

Essential Fatty Acids

Essential fatty acids cannot be manufactured by the body and must be supplied daily through the diet. Essential fatty acids are unsaturated fatty acids necessary for normal growth and healthy blood arteries, and nerves. Essential fatty acids are important for the transport and breakdown of cholesterol. They also keep skin and other tissues youthful and healthy. According to Udo Erasmus, author of "Fats and Oils," essential fatty acids are the highest source of energy in nutrition.

The three essential fatty acids are linolenic, linoleic, and arachidonic. Arachidonic fatty acids can be synthesized in the body if sufficient linoleic and linolenic are present.

Erasmus also tells us that one-third of our total fat intake should be essential fatty acids and the best sources are:

Flax seeds and flax seed oil

Soybeans and soybean oil

Sunflower, sesame, and pumpkin seeds and oil

Walnuts

Fish

Dark green vegetables, i.e.: Broccoli and spinach

To obtain essential fatty acids in the diet it is best to rely upon fresh, raw, unrefined foods or products like fresh, unrefined cold pressed oils.

How Much?

Lack of fats and essential fatty acids in the diet will cause a change in cell structure, resulting in slowed growth and other disorders. Symptoms include brittle and dull hair, nail problems, dandruff, allergies, and dermatitis, especially eczema in infants.

If too much fat is consumed, abnormal weight gain and obesity may result. Excessive fat intake will cause abnormally slow digestion and absorption, resulting in indigestion. If a lack of carbohydrates and water in the diet accompanies excess fat intake, fats cannot be completely metabolized and may become toxic to the body.

Recommendations for fat consumption range from 25-30 percent of total calorie intake. At least one-third of this should consist of the essential unsaturated fatty acids. The American Heart Association currently recommends that monunsaturated fats should take precedence over polyunsaturated fats in a 1.5 ratio to 1. Saturated fats should be avoided.

NOTE: Avoid prepared foods which often contain animal fat or tropical oils such as palm and coconut. These are often used because they are less expensive and produce aesthetically appealing products. To avoid saturated fats, manufactures often instead use hydrogenated or partially hydrogenated oils. Prepare your own foods as much as possible and **read labels carefully** before you buy anything!

One gram of fat yields approximately 9 calories to the body. According to the above recommendation:

A 160 pound man with calorie consumption of 2600 would require a fat intake of about 68 grams.

A 130 pound woman with calorie consumption of 2000 would require a fat intake of about 50 grams.

Following are a few food items and the approximate fat content they contain:

* One tablespoon butter:
100 calories
11.5 grams total fat
       7 grams saturated
       4 grams unsaturated
       31 milligrams cholesterol

* One glass whole milk
244 calories
8 grams total fat
5 grams saturated
3 grams unsaturated
33 milligrams cholesterol

* One ounce cheddar cheese
114 calories
9.4 grams total fat
5.98 grams saturated
2.93 grams unsaturated
30 milligrams cholesterol

* One ounce cream cheese
99 calories
9.89 grams total fat
6.23 grams saturated
3.15 grams unsaturated
31 milligrams cholesterol

* One tablespoon corn oil
120 calories
14 grams total fat
2 grams saturated
11 grams unsaturated
O cholesterol

* One tablespoon vegetable shortening
115 calories
12.8 grams total fat
5.2 grams saturated
7.1 grams unsaturated
0 cholesterol

* One cup peanuts
830 calories
70 grams total fat
14 grams saturated
50 grams unsaturated
0 cholesterol

* One avocado
324 calories
30.8 grams total fat
       4.9 grams saturated fat
       23.2 grams unsaturated
       0 cholesterol

* One 16 ounce T-bone steak
1600 calories
168 grams total fat
       70 grams saturated
       89 unsaturated
       261 milligrams cholesterol

* Two Ounce (One-eighth pound) bacon
315 calories
32 grams of total fat
       12 grams saturated
       19 grams unsaturated
       38 milligrams cholesterol

* One-third pound chicken (dark meat with skin)
125 calories
10 grams total fat
       2.5 grams saturated
       6 grams unsaturated
       43 milligrams cholesterol

* One-third pound chicken (white meat with skin)
72 calories
4.2 grams total fat
       1.3 grams saturated
       2.7 grams unsaturated
       29 milligrams cholesterol

* One-half pound pike
211 calories
2.7 grams total fat
       .38 grams saturated
       1 gram unsaturated

Fats to Avoid

Hydrogenated and partially hydrogenated fats are fats which have been changed from their natural liquid form to become more solid. These fats should be avoided because this processing alters the natural molecular structure of the fatty acids into an unnatural trans-configuration. These trans-fatty acids are unhealthy because they resemble saturated fats but the body has a much more difficult time processing them. Trans-fatty acids also produce free radicals in the body. Because very few amounts of trans-fatty acids occur in nature, they are "foreign" to the body.

Trans-fatty acids tend to raise Low Density Lipoprotein or LDL (undesirable) cholesterol levels and lower High Density Lipoprotein or HDL (desirable) cholesterol levels in the blood. In addition, these trans-fatty acids can easily become trapped along arterial walls creating an ideal environment for build-up of plaque and development of atherosclerosis.

In addtion, in such processing essential fatty acids are easily destroyed due to the presence of heat, oxygen and light.

Examples of hydrogenated fat products include margarine, margarine-based products, shortenings, and fats used for frying.

Butter vs Margarine

Butter contains easy-to-digest short-chain fatty acids, but contains relatively few essential fatty acids (only about 2 percent linoleic acid). Butter also contains about one gram cholesterol per pound of butter and does not contain the factors needed for its metabolism (oil seeds and fresh seed oils do contain these factors).

Butter contains fatty acid chains that are more easily metabolized than the fatty acid chains found in hydrogenated oils, fats, shortening and margarine. Butter can also be used for frying, baking, and heating because it consists mainly of saturated fats which are relatively stable in the presence of light, heat, and oxygen.

NOTE: Many commercial dairy's use antibiotics which can be found in butter and other dairy products. These can inflict allergies, tiredness, sugar craving, hypoglycemia and several other conditions.

Margarine does not contain much of the short-chain easily digestible fatty acids. The oil from which margarine is made does contain a substantial amount of unsaturated fatty acids but these are destroyed or changed into other substances in processing. Margarine contains less essential fatty acids than butter. The fatty acids it does contain are altered and interfere with the functions of essential fatty acids and often become concentrated in heart tissue. These fatty acids also are metabolized much slower than the ones in butter.

Margarine contains no cholesterol, but the metabolism of margarine still requires factors that have been refined.

Margarine contains no antibiotics or pesticides, but contains many other non-natural chemicals as a result of processing. The effect of these on health is yet unknown.

Margarine and other hydrogenated products are not good for cooking because the unsaturated fatty acids they do contain are further altered by heat, light and oxygen.

Margarine is advertised as the healthy choice, but the truth seems to be the opposite. Because of the way margarine is manufactured, it is actually more dangerous to one's health. Butter is more healthy in terms of digestibility, usefulness for frying and naturalness.

In addition, most people agree, butter tastes better, just don't over do it.

Did You Know...

The cheapest source of protein is found in beans?

For 60 grams (RDA) of protein, beans only cost about $ 0.33.

In comparison:

60 grams protein from peanut butter: $0.72
60 grams protein from milk: $0.84
60 grams protein from eggs: $0.78
60 grams protein from chicken: $0.96
60 grams protein from ground beef: $1.32
60 grams protein from American processed
    cheese: $1.41
60 grams protein from frankfurters: $1.77
60 grams protein from beef rump roast: $1.80
60 grams protein from ocean perch: $2.30
60 grams protein from bologna: $2.40
60 grams protein from veal: $5.55

PROTEIN

Next to water, protein is the most plentiful substance in the body. Proteins are a large group of complex, organic nitrogen compounds. Each are made up of linked amino acids that contain the elements carbon, hydrogen, nitrogen, and oxygen. Some proteins also contain sulphur, phosphorus, iron, iodine, or other necessary nutrients.

Protein is an important element for the maintenance of good health and vitality. Protein is the major source of material needed for the building and maintenance of muscles, skin, blood, hair, nails and internal organs, including the heart and brain. It is needed to make hormones and is vital to the maintenance of homeostasis, and other functions such as growth and rate of metabolism. Protein also helps prevent the blood and tissues from becoming too alkaline or acidic and helps regulate the body's water balance. Enzymes require protein as do antibodies, which help fight foreign substances in the body. Protein is necessary for proper release of body wastes.

Protein can also be a source of heat and energy providing four calories per gram. However, this energy function is spared when sufficient carbohydrates or fats are present in the diet. Excess protein that is not used for building tissues or energy can be converted by the liver and stored as fat in the body tissues.

Balance

An important aspect of obtaining a good diet is the balancing of amino acids. Twenty-two amino acids have been identified as necessary for growth, development and good health. The body requires these in a specific pattern in order to make human protein. The body can make 14 of these amino acids, called non-essential, while the other eight (essential) must be obtained from food. If just one

45

essential acid is missing, even temporarily, protein synthesis cannot continue. The result is that all amino acids are reduced in the same proportion as the amino acid that is low or missing.

Foods containing high amounts of protein are meat, poultry, fish, eggs, nuts, milk and cheese. Complete proteins have the eight essential amino acids. Complete proteins are usually found in foods of animal origin such as meats, poultry, seafood, eggs, milk and cheese.

Incomplete proteins are foods that lack or are extremely low in certain essential amino acids. These are not efficient when eaten alone. Nuts and legumes, including navy beans, chick peas, soybeans and split peas, are incomplete proteins since they do not contain all the essential amino acids. Fruits and vegetables may contain small amounts of protein, but are usually incomplete proteins. Mixing incomplete and complete protein sources can provide better nutrition than either one can alone.

For example, a rice (not white) and bean dish with some cheese can be just as nutritious, less expensive and lower in fat than a steak. Several vegetables can be combined together to make a complete protein. The amino acids missing in corn are ample in beans, thus the combination of tortillas and beans, a dietary staple of Central, South and some parts of North America, is an excellent source of high-quality, complete proteins.

NOTE: Some recent research indicates and some nutritionist believe the information claiming certain foods are incomplete proteins is outdated. Studies at the Max Planck Institute in Germany, one of the most respected nutrition research centers in the world, showed that many vegetable protein foods are "just as good or better than animal proteins." The vegetable foods said to be complete proteins are soybeans, peanuts, almonds, buckwheat, sunflower seeds, pumpkin seeds, potatoes, avocados, and all leafy green vegetables.

Also discovered and reported by the Max Planck Institute was raw proteins contained a higher biological value when compared to cooked proteins. Cooking makes all proteins less assimilable. It was suggested that one only needs about one-half the amount of proteins if only raw vegetable proteins are eaten instead of animal proteins, which are usually cooked.

How much?

Protein requirements differ according to each individual. Body stature, age, nutritional status, health, and physical activity will cause individual needs to vary. A body builder or other athlete in training would require a much larger amount of calories and therefore more protein. Stress, surgery, hemorrhage or prolonged illness will usually increase an individual's need for protein. It is critical that children get enough protein to reach their potential physical stature.

According to one source, the larger and younger you are, the more protein you require. To compute your personal daily needs, see chart below:

Age:	1-3	4-6	7-10	15-18	Over 19
Pound key:	.82	.68	.45	.40	.36

* Find the pound key under your age group.
* Multiply that number by your weight.
* The result will be your daily protein requirement in grams.

By this recommendation an 18 year old male who weighs 150 pounds would require 60 grams of protein.

Recommendations for protein intake are varied according to the various nutritionists. Recommendations usually vary between 10 to 20 percent, with the average around 15 percent of one's total calorie intake. Proteins yield about 4 calories per gram.

For example, according to this average of 15 percent:

A 160 pound man requiring 2600 calories daily would want to consume about 375 calories or 93 grams of protein.

A 130 pound woman requiring 2000 calories daily would want to consume about 300 calories or 75 grams of protein.

Listed below are several examples of foods containing protein:

* **One half chicken breast** (without skin)
  150 calories
  30 grams protein

* **Four ounces lean ground beef**
  200 calories
  23 grams protein

* **Four ounces cod**
  85 calories
  20 grams protein

* **One half cup navy beans**
  112 calories
  7.2 grams protein

* **One cup whole milk**
  150 calories
  8 grams protein

* **One half cup lowfat (2%) cottage cheese**
  110 calories
  15.5 grams protein

* **One ounce swiss cheese**
  107 calories
  8 grams protein

* **One large hard boiled egg**
  80 calories
  7 grams protein

* **One slice whole wheat bread**
  56 calories
  2.4 grams protein

* **One cup peanuts**
  830 calories
  30 grams protein

A protein deficiency can usually manifest in adults as poor muscle tone, hair and nails, lack of vigor and stamina, mental depression, weakness, poor resistance to infection, and slow healing of wounds and disease. Protein shortages among children can cause abnormal growth and certain diseases.

Excess protein intake may upset the body and cause several imbalances including fluid imbalance and can put a stress upon the kidneys. Excess protein, especially meat, can cause deficiencies of vitamins B-6 and B-3, because they are needed in abundance to metabolize proteins. These vitamins are not available from the meat itself and will be drawn from the body's own storage. Meat also contains 22 times more phosphorus than calcium. Because they are needed in about equal quantities in the diet, deficiencies of calcium and magnesium can result from excessive meat consumption. Phosphorus cannot be properly digested without calcium.

There are a variety of protein sources to choose from. Listed below are a few sources:

Meat

Meats conventionally are considered the most important source of complete protein. In addition to protein, beef, lamb, and pork are good sources of thiamine and riboflavin, phosphorus, iron, sulfur,

49

potassium, zinc, and copper. Poultry, also a good source of complete protein, contains several B vitamins (especially niacin), iron, and phosphorus.

The quality of beef, lamb, and pork is designated by the cut: Prime, Choice, or Good. The meat's flavor, tenderness, and ease of cooking vary with the grade and do not affect its nutritional value. Lean cuts with less fat are preferred. Prime and Choice cuts of meat are often not the highest in protein content because the meat contains larger amounts of marbling, or fat granules, to increase tenderness. Processed meats such as luncheon meats, bacon, frankfurters, and sausages are usually high in fats (and nitrates) and should be avoided.

Variety meats (liver, heart, etc.) are usually richer in vitamins and minerals than muscle meats. Liver is a very rich source of complete protein and B vitamins, especially riboflavin, niacin, and B-12. It is also a good source of vitamins A, C, and D, iron, phosphorus and copper. Organ meats are often high in cholesterol.

Fish

Fish is an excellent source of complete protein, polyunsaturated fatty acids, and minerals, especially iodine and potassium.

Fish are categorized as freshwater, saltwater and shell fish. Each type differs slightly in nutritive value. Freshwater fish contain magnesium, phosphorus, iron and copper. Saltwater and shellfish are rich in iodine, fluorine, and cobalt. High fat (10-15 percent) fish (salmon, sardines, mackerel, trout and eel) are good sources of vitamin A and D and provide the best sources of essential fatty acids. Herring, oysters, and sardines contain vanadium and zinc. Lean varieties of fish include halibut, sole, sea bass, and snapper. Shellfish are lower in essential fatty acids and higher in cholesterol.

Fresh fish is the healthiest, although it is also available frozen, canned, and dried. Dried foods can lose significant amounts of nutrients. Smoked and salted fish are not recommended. Smoking will decrease some of the nutrients, but this is not actually the reason it is not recommended. There are approximately 300 chemicals in smoke, many of which are classed as carcinogens by various health conscious individuals.

Fresh fish and shellfish should not remain at room temperature for more than two hours because of the possibility of bacterial infection. They should be well wrapped, stored in the coldest part of the refrigerator and used within two days. Fish and shellfish are best cooked at low temperatures and should not be overcooked, to preserve flavor, juices and nutrients.

Eggs

Eggs are an excellent source of complete protein. A large egg contains about seven or eight grams of protein. The protein in eggs is the most bioavailable and most compatible for humans because the protein structures are the most similar. Egg protein is very digestible and absorbable.

Eggs also contain vitamins A, B-2, D, and E, niacin, copper, iron, sulfur, phosphorus, selenium and essential fatty acids. The egg yolk contains lecithin which provides the richest known source of choline. Lecithin is necessary for keeping the cholesterol inside the egg emulsified. Egg yolk also contains biotin.

Eggs should be refrigerated at all times. A soiled egg should be wiped clean with a soft dry cloth instead of washed to preserve its natural protective film. This film prevents odors, flavors, molds, and bacteria from getting inside the egg. Eggs retain their freshness and quality better if stored large end up and in their original carton.
Raw eggs should not be consumed in large quantities. They contain avidin which interferes with the use of biotin and may also contain salmonella.

NOTE: The egg consumption in the United States is one half of what it was in 1945, yet there has not been a comparable decline in heart disease. Eggs do contain cholesterol, but they also contain lecithin and choline which aid in fat assimilation and raise high density lipoprotein (HDL) levels. The higher one's HDL levels, the lower one's chance of developing heart disease.

Legumes

Legumes are plants that have edible seeds within a pod. They include peas, beans, lentils, and peanuts. Legumes are a rich source of incomplete protein, fiber, iron, thiamine, riboflavin, and niacin.

Sprouting can increase the vitamin C content. Any enzyme inhibitors present will also be deleted if legumes are allowed to sprout. Because of their high but incomplete protein content, legumes can be used as a meat substitute when used with other complementary protein foods.

Dried legumes should be stored in tightly covered containers in a cool, dry place. They should be cooked in liquid to soften their cellulose fiber and to restore flavor and moisture lost in the drying process. Adding baking soda to speed up the softening process will destroy the thiamine content.

Nuts

Nuts are the dry fruits or seeds of some kinds of plants, usually of trees. Some readily available nuts are pecans, filberts, Brazil nuts, walnuts, almonds and cashews. The soft inside part of the nut is the meat, or kernel. The outer covering is the shell. Nuts contain high amounts of proteins, unsaturated fats, the B complex vitamins, vitamin E, calcium, iron, potassium, magnesium, phosphorus and copper.

Nuts that are shelled should be stored in airtight containers in the refrigerator to avoid any rancidity since they contain fat. If nuts are purchased in the shell, one should avoid ones with shells that are partially cracked because of rancidity.

Seeds

Seeds are the ripened ovules of plants. Edible seeds such as pumpkin seeds, sesame seeds, and sunflower seeds are rich in protein, the B complex vitamins, vitamins A, D and E, phosphorus, calcium, iron, fluorine, other minerals, and unsaturated fatty acids. Sunflower seeds contain up to 50 percent protein.

Other varieties of seeds used more for seasoning are poppy, caraway, dill, and anise.

Unhulled seeds have a long shelf life, provided kept covered in a cool dry place. Hulled seeds should be kept in the refrigerator and used immediately because the fat content causes them to spoil.

Milk and Milk Products

Dairy products are excellent sources of complete protein, calcium, and riboflavin. Milk also contains vitamins A, D, B-6, B-12, thiamine, phosphorus, and several other minerals. The fatty acids of milk are well balanced and supply saturated and unsaturated fat. According to Dr. Paava Airola, author of "Hypoglycemia: A Better Approach," dairy cholesterol has only a significant effect on the amount of cholesterol in the arteries and the excessive use of refined carbohydrates, such as white sugar and white flour, poses a much greater threat to the cholesterol levels in the body.

Milk is available in several forms: Raw, pasturized, homogenized, fermented and chesses. Pasteurizing milk will kill bacteria. The process involves heating milk to a high temperature and cooling it very rapidly. Unfortunately, many chemicals, hormones, and other fortification substances are often added in an attempt to restore what is destroyed during the heating process.

Homogenized milk has its fat content finely dispersed throughout, and is thought to be more easily digested. Many nutritionists recommend **fermented milk products** such as yogurt, kefir, acidophilus milk, piima, madzoon, buttermilk, or plain clobbered milk. These fermented, soured milks have approximately the same nutritive and health-building value (or more) and exceptional digestibility. Soured milks are superior to fresh milk because they are "predigested" and therefore, very easily assimilated.

NOTE: Avoid any of these products if sugar has been added.

Cheese is made by separating the curds (or milk solids) from the whey (or water part) of the milk. Its texture and flavor vary with ripening (aging). Most cheeses contain protein milk, fat, calcium, phosphorus, vitamin A, and riboflavin. Cheese should be stored in the refrigerator in its original container. There are many varieties of cheese; brick, cheddar, colby, cottage cheese, feta, limburger, mozzarella, parmesan, ricotta, and swiss are only a few of the many available. Varieties vary some in fat content, but most are excellent sources of complete protein. Avoid processed cheeses and cheese foods.

WATER

Water is the most abundant nutrient found in the body, accounting for about two-thirds of body weight. It is considered by many to be the most important nutrient because it is responsible for and involved in nearly every body process. It is commonly known that a person can live for weeks without food but only for a few days without water.

Water is involved in digestion, absorption, circulation, excretion, transport of nutrients, and is necessary for all building functions in the body. Water is the essential component of all cellular structure and is the medium in which all chemical reactions of cellular metabolism take place. Water also helps maintain a normal body temperature and is essential for flushing toxins out of the body.

The minerals in water are also very important for good health. Natural water is a very good source of chromium, a trace mineral that is vitally involved in sugar metabolism. Chromium is a co-factor with insulin, not only for sugar metabolism, but also for cholesterol metabolism and protein synthesis.

Drinking adequate water is the best treatment for fluid retention. When the body gets less water it perceives this as a threat and it begins to retain. Water is stored in the extracellular spaces (outside the cells). This shows up as swollen feel, legs, and hands. When you give the body the water it needs, the excess will be released.

Water helps to maintain proper muscle tone by giving muscles their natural ability to contract and by preventing dehydration.

Water can also help relieve constipation, When the body gets too little, it siphons what it needs from internal sources. The colon is one primary source. The result is constipation. With adequate water consumption, normal bowel function can return.

The average adult body contains about 45 quarts of water and loses about three quarts daily through respiration, excretion and perspiration. The rate of water loss depends almost entirely upon the levels of activity and the environment. A sedentary person in a normal climate may only lose one quart in a day while 10 quarts may be lost in a desert climate in one day. Severe deficiencies need to be corrected as soon as possible before salt depletion and dehydration advance and result in death.

Excess water may be lost from the body by profuse sweating, diarrhea, or prolonged episodes of vomiting.

Drinking eight eight ounce glasses of water daily is recommended for optimum health. This amount increases for those who are involved in athletic activities, in hot climates, are in ill health, or anything else causing increased perspiration.

The water available to us includes drinking water, the water present in liquids and juices, solid food consumed, and the water formed in the cells as a result of the oxidation of food consumed. Fruits and vegetables are especially good sources of chemically pure water, which is 100 percent pure hydrogen and oxygen.

Tap water is taken from streams, rivers and lakes. This water may contain pollutants and agricultural wastes, such as fertilizer and insecticide residues that are carried by rainwater runoff into nearby waterways. Air pollutants also end up in our rivers and streams. Because of this, chemicals are added to our tap water for purification purposes. Fluorine, chlorine, phosphates, alum, sodium aluminates, soda ash, carbon and lime are chemicals frequently added. These substances may be needed to kill bacteria but questions have been raised regarding the potential health hazards of many of these chemicals. Common industrial wastes in air pollution can combine with some of these chemicals producing carcinogenic substances. In a report to congress in 1975, data identified 253 different specific chemicals (such as pesticides and chloroform) in the drinking water in the United States.

In addition, if you are prone to allergies, fluorine, chlorine and many of these other additives may cause problems.

Hard tap water may contain high amounts of calcium and magnesium and other minerals that can irritate the colon and aggravate other undesirable symptoms individuals may have.

Well or spring water can also be polluted due to seepage of ground surface contaminants and the mineral content can vary extremely from one location to the next.

Distilled water is presumed to be the best type of water because distilling is the most efficient process to remove contaminants from the water. Distilled water, therefore, is highly recommended as drinking water for those wishing to avoid pollutants, chemicals and bacteria. For those who do drink distilled water, it is suggested that they also use mineral supplements because distilled water contains no minerals.

Natural mineral waters (provided they are uncarbonated) and sea water can also be used.

Part 2:
Ailments
and
Conditions

The following chapters provide information concerning common ailments and conditions. Not all of this information applies to each person suffering from the condition. Each causative factor, symptom and therapeutic regimen must be considered separately according to each individual.

Minor disorders in their early stages can usually be treated at home effectively and safely. Serious conditions may require attention from a medical professional. Although drugs and surgery are not advocated here, in some situations, they may be necessary.

ACNE

Acne is a common disorder of the skin characterized by recurring formation of pimples, whiteheads and blackheads. Acne breakouts usually occur on the face, shoulders and back where sebaceous oil glands are the most numerous and active. It is caused by clogging and inflammation of the oil gland and ducts beneath the skin. Acne affects about 75 percent of adolescent boys and 50 percent of adolescent girls.

Acne may occur as a result of inadequate diet (excessive saturated fat, hydrogenated fat, animal or dairy products, sugar and refined carbohydrates), nutritional deficiencies (particularly zinc and vitamin B-6), poor eliminations, build-up of toxins, and food allergies. Acne can be irritated by use of cosmetics and poor hygiene, stress, and monthly menstruation.

What to do:

* Wash daily with warm water.
* Do not irritate and contaminate infections by touching, or squeezing with your hands and fingers.
* To stop a flare-up when a pimple becomes visible, apply ice for a few seconds every 30 minutes. This should cause it to subside in a few hours. If it does not, apply a moist compress every hour.
* To take the red out of a blemish, combine one tablespoon of lemon juice with one tablespoon of salt. Apply this mixture to the red area and leave it on for 10 minutes and rinse.
* For mild to moderate cases of acne wash face at least three times daily with a mild, but effective hygiene soap. Soaps containing benzoyl peroxide should be avoided because they may be too harsh and may damage the skin.
* To get rid of a pimple overnight, dip a cotton swab in witch hazel or hydrogen peroxide and apply it to the

pimple to dry it up, then apply calamine lotion.

* Pimples will also heal faster if you put a drop of chamomile extract onto the blemish.

* Enemas or colon cleansing may be used to speed the toxins out of the body.

* Blood purifiers such as alfalfa, barberry, black cohosh, burdock, chaparral, dandelion, and red clover help clear toxins out of the blood and clear skin.

* Supplemental vitamin A has been effective in the treatment of acne. Topical use of the vitamin A from the capsule can also be effective.

* Supplemental zinc sulfate (150 mg total daily: 50 mg after each meal) has also proven to be very beneficial for the skin and has cured numerous conditions of acne-even severe cases. **NOTE:** If bowel upset occurs, reduce dosage and add one to three milligrams copper. Selenium also may be required at 100 micrograms daily.

* Increase intake of foods high in zinc:

> **Oysters** (160 mg zinc per four ounce serving)
> **Herring** (110 mg zinc per four ounce serving)
> **Wheat germ** (14 mg zinc per four ounce serving)
> **Sesame seeds** (10 mg per four ounce serving)
> **Torula yeast** (9.9 mg per four ounce serving)
> **Blackstrap molasses** (8.3 mg per four ounce serving)
> **Liver** (7 mg per four ounce serving)
> **Soybeans** (6.7 mg per four ounce serving)
> **Sunflower seeds** (6.6 mg per four ounce serving)
> **Egg yolk** (5.5 mg per four ounce serving)
> **Lamb** (5.4 mg per four ounce serving)

* Serious cases of acne may require medical attention because it may cause scarring.

Beneficial supplementation:

Vitamin A:
> *Therapeutic:* 50,000-100,000 IU daily for one month, then reduce dosage.
> *Maintenance:* 10,000-25,000 IU daily for one month, then reduce dosage. **Note:** (Beta carotene

is a safer source of vitamin A.)
Vitamin B Complex:
Vitamin B-6: 50-250 mg twice daily.
Niacin: 100 mg three times daily
Pantothenic Acid: 300 mg daily
Vitamin C:
  Therapeutic: 2,000 mg three to five times daily
  Maintenance: 1,000 mg three to four times daily
Vitamin D:
Vitamin E: (internal and topical)
Unsaturated Fatty Acids:
Calcium:
Potassium:
Sulfur: 1-30 grain daily
Zinc: 30-150 mg daily (zinc sulfate is commonly preferred)
Garlic: 2 capsules with meals
Lactobacillus acidophilus:
Herbs: Alfalfa, Aloe Vera (topical), Barberry, Black Cohosh, Blue Flag, Burdock, Chamomile (extract-topical), Chaparral, Chlorophyll, Coneflower, Dandelion, Echinacea, Oregon Grape, Red Clover, Valerian, and White Oak Bark.

How to avoid:

Good hygiene, adequate rest, exercise and sunlight are extremely important to the health of the skin.

Eating a proper diet plays a large role in the health of your skin. One should eat a balanced healthy diet low in saturated fat, low in refined sugar and simple carbohydrates, low in salt, and high in complex carbohydrates.

Zinc is anti-bacterial agent and a necessary element in the oil-producing glands of the skin. A diet low in zinc will trigger acne flare-ups. Be sure your diet provides adequate amounts of zinc. Foods rich in zinc include seafood, soybeans, whole grains, sunflower seeds and some nuts.

Avoid chocolate, cocoa, spinach, and rhubarb which

contain oxalic acid. Oxalic acid may inhibit the body's absorption of calcium which is needed to maintain the body's acid-alkaline balance of the blood. This is important for a clear complexion.

Avoid touching your face with your hands. for example resting your chin or forehead on your hand while sitting at a table. Hands, and fingers especially, are highly contaminated and a breeding ground for germs.

Acne flare-ups may be due to the use of cleansing creams, night moisturizers, face foundations and rouges. These products often contains additives such as fatty acids, coal tars and oils which can clog pores.

Also remember to wash make-up applicator brushes and sponges often to avoid contamination.

Avoid stress which can cause hormonal changes in the body and cause a acne flare-up.

AGING

Aging, although a natural process which is inevitable as we grow older, is accelerated with poor dietary habits and abuse to the body.

As we grow older, research shows that because of changes in metabolism and the conversion of food to energy, there is an increase in the daily requirements of a number of important nutrients. According to some authorities, the RDAs in their present form may actually result in insufficiencies of certain nutrients leading to increased risk to later stage diseases. An increased risk for these conditions is a direct result of suboptimal nutrition. Many conditions, known as "old-age" diseases, are not necessarily old-age diseases, but diseases of the consequence of suboptimal nutrition consumed over a period of time which increased the risk for these conditions later in life.

Recognition is growing that specific nutrients such as vitamins B-6, B-12, C, D, and E and the minerals calcium, zinc, iron and chromium are required in significantly larger mounts as we grow older to optimize function.

Cross-linking is a term commonly associated with aging of the skin. It refers to the bonds which hold the outer surface skin cells together. As you grow older, these bonds become more cross linked and stronger. The cells do not shed as easily as they did when you were younger. The outermost layer of skin cells therefore becomes "older" and thicker causing a leathery look.

Cross-linking at the molecular level causes skin (and body) to be less agile. Cross-linking can occur at all levels of cell functions, including the nucleic acids, DNA and RNA, which are the master instructors of the cell. In this case, the cells cannot function properly and abnormal cells result.

Cross-linking is caused by a chemical acetaldehyde, found in cigarette smoke and smog and made in the liver from alcohol; and by free radicals, which are created by radiation and the oxidation of fats. Free radicals damage proteins, fats, and DNA and RNA. Free radicals also cause brownish pigments in the skin called age spots.

Free radicals are highly reactive chemicals believed to be the cause of destruction and death in nearly all living things. Free radicals occur when healthy oxygen molecules are transformed into a highly reactive, unstable form of oxygen. This transformation occurs ironically by things we trust most like sunlight, the air we breath, the food we eat and things we do everyday, like exercise.

Compounded by environmental pollution, food additives, cured meats, tobacco smoke, alcohol, infection, stress, chemotherapy, asbestos, X-rays, pesticides, and other manmade pollutants, free radicals can multiply at an alarming rate.

Free radicals can attack, damage and ultimately destroy any material, not just the sensitive cells and tissues of the skin and inside the body. Free radicals degrade collagen and reprogram DNA and are implicated in more that 60 diseases, including Alzheimer's, Parkinson's, cancer, arthritis, cataracts, kidney and liver disorders.

To prevent such damage, free radical molecules must be scavenged and destroyed by antioxidants. Antioxidants "blanket" the activity of free radicals, preventing them from damaging cells and preventing the spread of further damage.

Free-radical damage can also occur in the liver causing it to age faster and making it function less than optimal.

Sunshine is the most harmful influence to your skin. Years of exposure to the sun exaggerates and accelerates one's natural aging process. It is the primary cause of premature aging; causing wrinkling, thinning of the skin, and the appearance or darkening of brownish discolorations known as "age spots," and broken blood vessels. Sunshine accelerates the normal loss of moisture and elasticity of the skin. Twenty years of sunning can leave you looking 15 to 20 years older than you really are. In addition, the sun is the primary cause of skin cancer.

Because of its external exposure, the skin is subject

to aging faster than our other organs. The epidermis is greatly affected by external factors, both good and bad. The dermis is only affected by internal factors, again, good and bad. The skin, especially the epidermis, is vulnerable to wear and tear, and therefore, unlike our other organs in the body (provided we do not abuse them), is not maintenance free.

When the skin begins to age, the following occurs:

1. **The skin becomes thinner.**
2. **Fewer skin cells are produced.**
3. **Skin cells grow more slowly.**
4. **The outermost layer (stratum corneum) becomes less effective for protection.**
5. **The skin retains less water.**
6. **Blood vessels become fewer.**
7. **Sweat and oil gland activity decreases leading to dryness and itching.**
8. **Collagen and elastin fibers become more rigid, causing the skin to wrinkle and sag.**

In the outermost layer of skin, the first signs of aging are dryness and cellular build-up.

Wrinkles appear when the action lines of the face deepen to form a crease in the skin. Loss and redistribution of fat tend to emphasize sagging and wrinkles. Wrinkles will usually appear first where the skin is the most thin, such as around the eyes and eyelids, the neck, and jaw lines. Eventually, jowls develop, the neck becomes creased, lines begin to radiate from the mouth, and "crow's feet" and "bags" develop around the eyes.

In addition, the pores of the skin will look larger, the skin will lose its water-holding ability and the dry cells will tend to curl up causing a rough, blotchy look.

In the inner layer of skin, the contour and color tone of the skin are lost with aging. When the inner layer deteriorates, the elastic elastin and collagen fibers become more rigid, less elastic and can even break into small pieces. Thus, effectiveness is lost which results in the outer surface collapsing, causing deep wrinkles and lines. The skin around the eyes and neck are the most vulnerable. Changes usually first appear in these areas where sagging is first obvious.

Also, in the inner layer of skin, newer cells are produced more slowly and older cells are repaired less effectively. Sweat and oil gland activity decreases with age contributing to dry skin associated with aging. This problem is usually worse for women than it is for men. One function of the oil glands is to manufacture and secrete oil to the surface of the skin where it acts as a natural barrier to prevent water loss through evaporation. The oil does not serve to moisturize the skin, it merely helps hold in the moisture you already have.

Dry skin contributes to skin problems by scaling, cracking, eczema, irritation, and infection. Dryness of the skin also accentuates existing wrinkles, making them look deeper and more abundant.

What to do:

* Preventative nutrition is the best defense against mental and physical aging. The diet should include natural unprocessed foods which contain adequate amounts of all essential nutrients. Supplementation is recommended in most cases.

* A diet very high in bromelain (pineapple) and papain (papaya) seems to help offset the normal negative effects from the sun.

* Damage from free radicals can greatly be reduced by taking antioxidants such as vitamins A, C, E, B-1, B-5, B-6, beta carotene, bioflavonoids (such as pycnogenol and activated quercetin), zinc, selenium, and the amino acids cysteine and glutathione.

* Catalyst Altered Water has antioxidant properties to help fight against free-radical damage and may be consumed or used topically.

* Vitamin E is known fairly well to protect the body against cellular aging.

* Because aging effects RNA synthesis, which is associated with memory storage, RNA supplements may be taken. Fish, especially sardines, is a good source of RNA. Chlorella is one of the best sources of vegetative of RNA and DNA. **NOTE:** In the body, metabolism of RNA

can form uric acid. Individuals who are susceptible to gout attacks may wish to substitute vitamin B-12 which stimulates natural RNA synthesis in the body.

Suggested Supplementation:

Vitamin A:
Beta Carotene (including marine carotenes):
Vitamin B-1
Vitamin B-3 (niacin):
Vitamin B-5:
Vitamin B-6:
Vitamin B-12:
Vitamin C:
Vitamin D:
Vitamin E:
Bioflavonoids:
Chromium:
Iron:
Selenium:
Zinc:
Cysteine:
Protein:
Papain and bromelin:
RNA:
Herbs: Alfalfa, Damiana, Dong Quai, Garlic,
    Ginseng, Gotu Kola, Pau D'Arco, and Red Clover.

How to Avoid:

Eat three sensible, well-balanced meals daily (low in fat and high in complex carbohydrates).

Substitute meat protein with soy. Soy provides complete protein nutrition. Soy milk is nutritious, good tasting, requires no refrigeration and can be stored indefinitely.

Substitute vegetables for meat and dairy products.

Substitute fish for meat as often as possible. Fish contains oils that may prevent heart attacks. Heart disease is the number one cause of death in America.

Eat bulk (high fiber) foods.

Cut down or avoid sugar and chemical additives to food.

Increase your intake of beta carotenes such as carrots, spinach, broccoli, and cantaloupe. Beta carotene has been shown to be protective against cancer. Cancer is the number two cause of death in America.

Stay on a basic low-fat diet to prevent heart disease and cancer. Avoid saturated fat (i.e. tropical oils) and hydrogenated oils. Read labels before buying and make ingredient inquiries when eating out. !

Use fish oils, flax seed oil and olive oil in salads and cooking. Research has shown that these oils lower cholesterol.

Avoid fried foods.

Keep your caloric intake and weight low to help slow aging.

To help keep body tissues healthy eat more foods high in vitamin C (citrus fruit, green vegetables, green peppers, etc.).

Eat foods high in vitamin E (vegetable oils and grains), zinc (pork, pumpkin seeds), and selenium (bran, tuna, fish).

Use charcoal or some other water filtering device to help eliminate chlorine and cancer-causing materials from your water or drink distilled water.

Avoid alcoholic beverages or drink only in moderation.

Do not smoke and avoid others that smoke.

Exercise regularly. Walking, swimming, or gardening are good.

Get seven to eight hours of sleep each night.

Eliminate stress.

Get fresh air every day if possible.

Use laughter to banish anxiety and fear. Let everyday be joyous.

Have a fresh, optimistic outlook on life!

Finally to prevent aging of the skin: Avoid the sun, avoid the sun, and avoid the sun! Use a minimum of SPF 15, especially on the face, if you are going to be outdoors. Wear a hat and protective clothing.

ALCOHOLISM

Alcoholism is a dependence on or an addiction to alcohol. Alcohol is a depressant which decreases the basic speed of all bodily functions. Heavy alcohol use can cause hepatitis, cirrhosis of the liver, gastritis (painful inflammation of the stomach lining), neuritis (inflammation of the nerves), damage to the brain and vitamin deficiencies.

Alcohol is a carbohydrate but contains no vitamins or minerals which are needed for carbohydrate metabolism. Therefore vitamins and minerals, especially the B-complex, vitamin C, zinc, magnesium, etc., are then taken from other parts of the body, and are readily depleted. In addition, vitamins A, B-1 (thiamine), B-2 (riboflavin), B-6, B-12, D, folic acid, and calcium are lost.

Complications and symptoms of alcoholism include food allergies, blackouts, dizziness, slurred speech, incoordination, nervousness, irritability, tremors, heart disease, liver disease, increased cholesterol levels, high blood pressure, and blood sugar disorders.

Alcoholism can be triggered by poor diet, ("high carbohydrate junk food diet" consisting of refined foods, excess sugar, vitamin and mineral deficiencies- especially B Complex, and excess coffee), hypoglycemia, stress, psychological addiction, and heredity.

What to do:

* Avoid over-indulgence and if symptoms of alcoholism occur or alcohol is consumed to a point where it interferes with the performance of daily activities, avoid alcohol completely. One may require counseling or outside assistance, such as Alcoholics Anonymous for support.

* To help prevent a hangover, take a B-Complex before going out, while you are drinking and in the

73

morning to help replace the B vitamins lost while drinking. **NOTE:** Vitamin B-1 deficiency (beriberi) is very common in the late stages of alcoholism.

* Vitamin C intravenously (20-30 grams daily) can help reduce withdrawal symptoms.

* To aid in recovery of alcoholism one requires a stable blood sugar level: Eliminate refined carbohydrates, especially white sugar and white flour, maintain a diet high in protein, and note suggested supplementation below.

* Selenium helps protect against alcohol-induced liver damage.

* Because alcohol is a diuretic, drink water while you are drinking and afterwards to replenish lost fluids.

* Two tablespoons of Swedish bitters is a fast-acting sobering tonic.

To reduce cravings for alcohol:

* Vitamin B-3 (Niacin) and the amino acid glutamine have been shown to help prevent the craving for alcohol. These supplements may be helpful. Glutamine also decreases the harmful poisoning effects of alcohol.

* The herb angelica is beneficial to induce a distaste for alcohol.

* Avoid coffee.

* Avoid non-nutrient "junk foods," which tend to increase cravings for alcohol.

* Supplement B Complex vitamins.

Beneficial supplementation:

Vitamin A (preferably beta carotene): 25,000-50,000
    IU daily
B Complex: 50-1,500 mg 3 times daily
Vitamin B-1: 100-300 mg daily
Vitamin B-3: 100 mg - 6 grams daily
Vitamin B-6: 50-100 mg twice daily
Vitamin C: 3-10 grams daily
Vitamin D: 1,000 IU
Vitamin E: 1,000 IU

74

Chromium: 200 mcg daily
Iron:
Magnesium: 1,000 mg
Manganese: 50 mg
Selenium: 200 mcg daily
Zinc: 150 mg
Glutamine: 1,000 IU two to three times daily
Brewer's Yeast: One teaspoon three times daily
Raw liver tablets:
Herbs: Alfalfa, Angelica, Cayenne, Goldenseal,
Valerian, Skullcap, Chaparral, Hops, Red Clover,
and Swedish Bitters.

Did You Know...

Sprouted potatoes can make you sick? Sprouted potatoes may contain elevated levels of natural nerve toxins called glycoalkaloids. If ingested, this can cause drowsiness, headache, diarrhea and high blood sugar. Always store potatoes in a cool, dark place. If they sprout, peel at least one-eighth inch into the flesh before cooking. Always remove the eyes and spouts.

NOTE: Baked potatoes contain safer levels of glycoalkaloids than fried potatoes.

ALLERGIES

An allergy is a sensitivity to some particular substance known as an allergen. An allergen can be a food, an inhalant such as pollen, mold, dust, animal dander or hair, an insect sting, chemicals, and a number of additional types. Most allergens are protein in nature. An allergic reaction may be hay fever (watery eyes, runny nose, sinus stuffiness, etc.), asthma, hives, eczema, high blood pressure, abnormal fatigue, abnormal hunger, stomach cramps, vomiting, anxiety, depression and other mental disorders, constipation, stomach ulcers, dizziness, headache, hyperactivity, insomnia, hypoglycemia, etc. Allergies are often difficult to detect, for example, an individual who suffers from reoccuring colds may actually be suffering from an unidentified food allergy.

Susceptibility to an allergen depends on heredity and the condition of one's immune system. Stress and hypoglycemia (adrenal exhaustion), poor diet (Vitamins C and B Complex deficiency), high copper levels, inadequate sleep, poor eliminations, emotional trauma, and infection can weaken the immune system making one more susceptible to an allergic reaction.

What to do:

* If possible, remove and avoid the allergen. Live in a clean environment: Vacuum carpets and rugs daily, change vacuum bags frequently, dust daily with oil-treated cloth so you do not spread the dust around, enclose your pillow and box spring in a plastic to reduce dust and dust mites, and avoid aerosol sprays and other irritating substances.

* Keep bedroom free of objects that collect dust, such as carpet, books, stuffed animals, etc. If possible get an air purifier or negative ion generator, especially for the bedroom.

* Avoid opening windows, if possible get an air

77

conditioner for your home. **NOTE:** It is crucial that you clean the filter on your air conditioner at least once a week to avoid buildup of mold and dust.

* Watercress is an old folk remedy for traditional allergy symptoms: Sneezing, stuffy head and watery eyes.

* Try to identify food allergies so that you can avoid those foods with the rotation diet or the pulse test.

* Avoid foods which have many ingredients such as commercial bread, catsup or salad dressing. Hidden ingredients in canned and packaged foods can undo an non-allergenic diet. Many authorities recommend eating no processed foods.

* Vitamin C is essential to adrenal function, acts as an antihistamine and antioxidant.

* Vitamin E has also shown to reduce histamine levels in the blood.

* B Complex vitamins, especially B-6, are essential for adrenal function.

* Vitamin B-5 is essential for cortisone production and acts as an antihistamine.

* Supplement hydrochloric acid and digestive enzymes. A slow down in production of these occurs in individuals in their forties, fifties, sixties, etc.

* Ma Huang (chinese ephedra), a natural anti-histamine, can be used as needed or on a regular basis.

* Colostrum, which contains immune-regulatory factors, as well as other vital immune support nutrients, may be benefiicial because allergies are concidered an immune disfunction disorder. **NOTE:** If you have allergies in your family history and become pregnant, it is of critical importance that you breast-feed your infant to ensure optimal immune development.

Beneficial supplementation:

Vitamin A: 10,000-25,000 IU
B-Complex: 25-50 mg three times daily
Vitamin B-5 (Pantothenic Acid): 100-200 mg
Vitamin C: 3-20+ grams daily to saturation level
Bioflavonoids:

Vitamin D:
Vitamin E:
Calcium:
Magnesium:
Manganese:
Molybdenum:
Selenium:
Zinc:
Colostrum: 1,000 mg three to four times daily.
Bee Pollen: (start at small doses and gradually build up.)
Digestive Enzymes:
Hydrochloric acid:
Raw adrenal tablets:
Herbs: Alfalfa, Burdock, Comfrey, Echinecea, Golden Seal, and Ma Huang (Chinese ephedra).

ANOREXIA NERVOSA

Anorexia nervosa is an eating disorder that usually strikes younger women who suppress the urge to eat to the point of malnutrition and starvation. Anorexia is characterized by broken blood vessels in the face, underweight, weakness, and dizziness.

In contrast, bulimia is constant excessive insatiable appetite followed by self-induced vomiting. Both anorexia and bulimia may be symptoms of a disease and/or psychotic problems.

What to do:

* Zinc has been 80 percent successful in aiding anorexic individuals regain appetite and gain weight. When the anorexic stops eating, zinc levels drop. As zinc levels in the body go down, the sense of smell and taste is destroyed. Without these senses, the desire for food decreases further.
* Supplementation is crucial to help prevent malnutrition.
* Counseling may be necessary.

Beneficial supplementation:

Vitamin A:
B Complex: 50 mg with each meal
Vitamin C:
Bioflavonoids:
Vitamin D:
Vitamin E:
Calcium:
Magnesium:
Potassium:
Sodium:
Zinc:

Free-form amino acids

Herbs: Chamomile, Dandelion, Kelp, Ladies Slipper, Licorice, Passion Flower, Skullcap, Red Clover, Wild Yam, and Yellow dock.

ARTHRITIS

Arthritis is a degenerative condition involving inflammation of the joints marked by pain and swelling. The cause of arthritis is not totally understood. It is thought to be related to the immune system (autoimmunity) or to nutritional deficiencies (excess meat and soda drinks, excess refined carbohydrates (sweets), raw vegetable deficiency, excess acid-forming foods, and excess vitamin D. Poor eliminations, glandular imbalances, psychological factors, lack of exercise, excess copper blood levels, and excess irritants (coffee, tea, salt, spices, alcohol) are additional etiologic considerations.

Some authorities suggest that arthritis may be induced by the intake of too much calcium and by taking the wrong forms of calcium. The calcium migrates to the soft tissues and deposits there. The tissues become calcified and the cells cease to function normally.

The two main types of arthritis are osteoarthritis and rheumatoid arthritis.

Osteoarthritis develops as a result of the continuous wearing away of cartilage in a bone. Osteoarthritis usually affects the weight-bearing joints such as the hips and knees of elderly individuals. Onset of osteoarthritis is gradual, with progressive pain and joint enlargement. It may involve single or multiple joints, but does not migrate from joint to joint.

Rheumatoid arthritis affects the whole body instead of just one joint. Synovial membrane (connective tissue) thickens and joint swells with redness and tenderness. Symmetrical joint involvement is common. Pain may migrate from joint to joint. Subcutaneous nodules are commonly found. Onset is abrupt or insidious. Onset of the disease may be related to physical or emotional stress, or may be poor nutrition or a bacterial infection.

Warning signs of arthritis:
* Swelling in one or more joints
* Early morning stiffness
* Unexplained weight loss, fever, or weakness combined with joint pain.
* Recurring pain or tenderness in any joint
* Obvious redness and warmth in a joint.

What to do:

* A diet of no red meat, white flour, white sugar, salt, citrus fruits, and /or nightshade family (tomatoes, potatoes, green pepper, eggplant) is helpful for relief of arthritis.

* Magnesium supplementation will help keep calcium in solution in the body. Some authorities recommend a 2:1 ratio of magnesium to calcium.

* Silica and potassium are important because silica will convert to calcium if needed.

* Vitamin C is useful because it increases natural cortisone production which is anti-inflammatory and helpful to the adrenals. Large doses may aggravate some cases, so be careful to evaluate its effect separately from other medications. Try ascorbate form of vitamin C if this is a problem.

* Niacinamide increases joint mobility by 85 percent if taken daily for three to four weeks. It is especially beneficial for osteoarthritis, although rheumatoid arthritis can also benefit. If nausea occurs, reduce dosage.

* SOD (Super Oxide Dismutase), a powerful natural antioxidant has been proven effective for rheumatoid arthritis when injected. Reliable SOD tablets also have proven effective when taken orally. **NOTE:** Green Barley Juice tablets are a good source of SOD.

* Low homeopathic doses of bryonia are useful for pain aggravated by movement.

* Colostrum, which contains immune-regulatory factors, as well as other vital immune support nutrients, may be benefiicial because arthritis is concidered an auto-immune disorder.

* Get at least 10-12 hours of rest each day, including naps.

* Avoid fatigue by splitting up big jobs and resting in intervals.

* Do not skip prescribed exercises-even if you have a painful flare-up.

* Use "contrast baths" for aching hands and feet...place them in warm water for three minutes, then cold water for one minute.

* Respect your pain. If a joint becomes painful for several hours after an activity, do not repeat the activity.

* Castor oil packs (see appendix) may be useful for correct eliminations.

Beneficial supplementation:

Vitamin A: 25,000-50,000 IU daily
B Complex: (extra B-6, B-12)
Niacinamide: 200-2,000 mg two to four times daily
Vitamin C: 3,000 -10,000 mg
Bioflavonoids: 3,000 mg
Vitamin E: 600-1,000 IU
Calcium: 800-1,000 mg daily
Magnesium: 400-800 mg daily
Potassium:
Selenium:
Sulphur:
Zinc: 25-50 mg one to two times daily
Protein:
Colostrum: 1,000 mg four or more times daily
DL Phenylalanine: 300 mg three times daily
Bromelain enzymes: Two to four tablets three times
    daily
Unsaturated Fatty Acids:
Cod Liver Oil: Three to four capsules daily
SOD:
Raw adrenal tablets:
Raw thymus tablets:
Herbs: Alfalfa, Devil's Claw, Echinacea, White Willow,
    and Yucca.

Did You know...

One dill pickle contains only 11 calories, but 1,426 mg of sodium?

ASTHMA

Asthma is a chronic respiratory condition characterized by difficulty in breathing, coughing and feeling of suffocation. Attacks can last for several minutes or several days.

An asthma attack may be triggered by an allergen, irritants, emotions, low blood sugar, or disorders of the adrenal glands. Asthma may be associated with diet (excess carbohydrates and sweets, excess dairy products, and overeating), food additives (especially sulfites), and poor eliminations.

Asthma is also commonly caused by cervical and thoracic spinal lesions.

What to do:

* Vitamin C has been shown to help control asthma when taken on a daily basis. Vitamin C acts as a natural antihistamine and antioxidant.

* Vitamin B-6 is also a natural antihistamine which is beneficial to help control asthma.

* Coffee which contains caffeine has been shown to relieve asthma symptoms. Caffeine equivalent to two cups of coffee unclogged blocked bronchial passages.

* In emergencies, Ma Huang, which contains ephedrine, is very useful as a bronchodilator.

* Asthma weed is useful for most asthmatics. Use 25 drops tincture in a small amount of water two to four times daily.

* Bee pollen is helpful as a preventative to inhalant allergies.

* If possible remove element which triggered the attack.

* During an attack try to remain as calm as possible and concentrate on your breathing.

* Visualization and meditation can be helpful to slow down your breathing.

* Concentrate on your breathing. Breath from the diaphragm.

* During an attack, it also may be beneficial to hold onto something above your head so that your arms are raised.

* Blood purifiers and colon cleansers may also be beneficial when used on occasion.

Beneficial supplementation:

Vitamin A:
> *Children:* 10,000 IU two to four times daily in acute cases.
> *Adults:* Up to 75,000 IU daily in acute cases

B Complex:
> *Children:* 25 mg three times daily.
> *Adults:* 50 mg three times daily

Vitamin B-5: 100 mg

Vitamin B-6: 100-250 mg twice daily

Vitamin C: 1,000-10,000 mg daily

Bioflavonoids:

Vitamin D: 1,000 IU daily

Vitamin E: 600 IU daily (32 IU for children)

Calcium: 400-1,000 mg daily (in acute cases, take every half hour)

Magnesium: 200-500 mg daily

Manganese: 5 mg two times per week

Potassium:

Molybdenum:

Zinc: 15-25 mg two to three times daily

Bee Pollen: Start at low dosages and build up gradually

Garlic: Two capsules daily with meals

Raw adrenal tablets: One tablet two to three times daily

Herbs: Alfalfa, Asthma Weed, Capsicum, Chlorophyll, Cascara Sagrada, Comfrey, Fenugreek, Garlic, Hops, Licorice, Ma Huang (ephedra), and Slippery Elm.

How to avoid:

There are a number of common triggers for an attack which should be avoided if possible. These include:
Extremely cold air
Excessive humidity
Air pollution
Tobacco smoke
Perfume or cologne fumes
Fumes from paint, paint thinner, chlorine bleach, etc.
Exercise
Infections caused by viruses
Stress or emotions (anger, fear, excitement, etc.)
Laughing
Pollen, mold, spores, animal dander, hair,
    feathers, etc.
Certain foods such as chocolate, nuts, eggs, etc.
Sulfites (commonly found in restaurant salads,
    and salad bars, frozen shrimp, potatoes, baked
    goods, sausage and wines, dairy products, white
    sugar and white flour products)
Other foods to avoid:
Sweets
Refined foods
Excessive carbohydrates
Excessive wheat and dairy products
Additives
Alcohol, tea, or other non-food irritants
Very hot and very cold foods

BACK PAIN

Backache may be a symptom of a variety of disturbances in the muscles, tendons, ligaments, bones, or underlying organs, for example, kidney infection. Backache could be the result of constipation, back strain, stress or calcium deficiency.

What to do:

The best self-help therapies for acute-low back pain include bed rest, cold therapy, acupressure, posture realignment, and stress reduction. You may need to know the exact cause of the pain before you can apply proper treatment. If pain so indicates, a visit to your physician or chiropractor may be necessary. For pain relief, phenylalanine may be used.

Beneficial supplementation:

B complex:
Niacin:
Vitamin C:
Vitamin D:
Vitamin E:
Calcium:
Magnesium:
Manganese:
Phosphorus:
Zinc:
Protein:
Phenylalanine:
Herbs: Alfalfa, Comfrey, Horsetail, Oatstraw, and
    Slippery Elm.

How to avoid:

Keep your weight down.Do not smoke.

Exercise to build strong back and stomach muscles.

Avoid standing or sitting in one position for a long period of time.

While on the phone, do not hold the receiver between your shoulder and head for long periods.

Wear comfortable shoes. The higher the heel, the greater the risk of backache.

When carrying things on your shoulder, switch the weight to your other shoulder from time to time.

When lifting, keep you back straight and bend your knees letting your knees do most of the work.

Always push large objects, never pull them.

Sleep on a firm mattress.

The worst sleeping position for your back is flat on your stomach with the head raised on a pillow. If you sleep on your stomach, place a pillow under your abdomen to raise your back slightly.

You can rest your back by lying on your side and pulling your knees towards your chin.

While sitting down, keep your knees about an inch higher that your hips to reduce strain on the back muscles.

Use a slant board regularly.

BAD BREATH

Bad breath (halitosis) can be caused by poor oral hygiene, nose or mouth infection, tonsillitis, tooth and gum decay, constipation, smoking or the presence of foreign bacteria. Diabetes, nervous tension, chemicals such as arsenic, lead, bismuth, and methane, or buildup of heavy metals, may also be the cause of bad breath.

Usually, bad breath is attributed to putrefactive bacteria living in undigested food which release gas through expelled air.

What to do:

* Brush your teeth, tongue, and floss your teeth.

* Change your toothbrush often where bacteria can hide and be reinoculated into the mouth.

* Store your toothbrush in a solution of hydrogen peroxide to kill microorganisms.

* Use a mouthwash containing zinc. The source of most mouth odor is sulphur compounds. A zinc containing mouthwash will negate these compounds for at least three hours. Zinc is also antibacterial.

* Try chewing celery or carrots which help rid the teeth of bacteria and make the mouth cleaner.

* Avoid excessive consumption of carbohydrates which can cause tooth decay.

* Supplement your diet with Lactobacillus acidophilus, also known as "friendly bacteria." Bad breath is often associated with putrefactive bacteria living on undigested food in the stomach. This condition causes gas to be released through the breath. Supplementing the diet with the friendly bacteria acidophilus often helps.

* Supplement chlorophyll, "Nature's Deodorant," which helps remove heavy metal poisons and sweetens the breath.

Beneficial supplementation:

Vitamin A: (Important for the all around health of the mouth.)

Niacin:

Zinc: 50 mg three times daily

Lactobacillus acidophilus: 1-2 tbsp liquid one to three times daily or one to two capsules two times daily.

Multiple digestive enzyme tablet: One three times daily

HCL:

Charcoal:

Bran or other fiber: One teas. with water before meals.

Chlorophyll:

How to avoid:

Avoid "bad breath" foods: Meat, stringy vegetables, sweets and especially sticky sweets.

Maintain good oral hygiene by brushing after each time you eat.

BALDNESS

Baldness is the partial or complete loss of hair (scalp), resulting from heredity, hormonal factors, aging, mineral deficiencies, poor circulation, medications, sluggish thyroid, or local or systemic diseases.

Stress, triggering a hormonal imbalance that over produces androgen, a male hormone, can cause both male and female pattern baldness. Male pattern baldness comprises a majority of hair loss causes.

What to do:

* Cayenne pepper, which has a stimulatory effect on cells, when rubbed into the scalp has resulted in regrowth of hair.
* Eliminate white sugar and white flour products.
* Use a blood purifier.
* Try hair shampoos containing caprylic acid.
* Use a slant board regularly.
* Make sure you get adequate protein in the diet, a major component of hair.

Beneficial supplementation:

Vitamin A:
B Complex:
Vitamin B-6: 50 mg
Choline: 500-1,000 mg
Folic Acid: 1 mg
Inositol: 500-1,000 mg
Niacin: 50 mg
PABA: 50-3,000 mg
Pantothenic Acid: 50 mg
Vitamin C: 1,000 mg
Vitamin E: 1,200 IU
Bioflavonoids: 50-100 mg

Copper:
Calcium:
Magnesium:
Manganese:
Potassium iodine:
Iron:
Silicon:
Sulphur:
Zinc:
Protein
L-Methionine: (Take with Vitamins B-6 and C for
    proper absorption.)
Raw thyroid:
Herbs: Aloe Vera, Horsetail, Jojoba, Kelp, and
    Oatstraw.

How to avoid:

Inositol and PABA protect hair follicles, preventing hair loss and often premature graying.

Biotin may slow hair loss.

BODY ODOR

Body odor is related not only to hygiene, but also to the inner health of the body. Certain nutrients (magnesium, zinc, vitamins B-6 and PABA) appear to metabolically remove wastes in the body which cause odors. An overdose of vitamin B-1 can cause odor in some people.

What to do:

* Many people suffer body odor despite good hygiene. magnesium taken with zinc, PABA, and vitamin B-6 can help control odors.
* Daily washing may be unnecessary and can actually wash away natural body oils that lubricate and protect the skin from bacteria.
* Avoid commercial deodorants that prevent perspiration because they clog the skin and prevent waste products from leaving the body.
* Supplement Burdock which restores oil and sweat gland functioning.

Beneficial supplementation:

B Complex:
Vitamin B-6:
PABA:
Magnesium:
Zinc: 20-40 mg
Essential Fatty Acids:
Chlorophyll: "Nature's deodorant"

Did You Know...

Non-stick pans may be dangerous? Non-stick pans such as Teflon (TM) or Silverstone (TM) can be dangerous if allowed to boil dry. At 400 degrees Fahrenheit, the pans may release toxic fumes after 20 minutes-enough to make a person sick. Pets, especially birds, are even more susceptible.

BRUISES

Bruises are caused from breaks in the small blood vessels in the soft tissue beneath the skin. These breaks leak blood which cause a reddish mark on the surface of the skin. This bruise turns blue then yellow as the blood is gradually absorbed.

Factors which make one susceptible to bruising are being overweight, anemia, time of menstrual period, lack of vitamins D, C, bioflavonoids, or zinc. Too much aspirin can also cause bruising.

What to do:

* DMSO, applied externally, may prevent the discoloration of bruises. DMSO acts as a scavenger of free radicals that are produced when blood vessels are damaged.

* The antioxidants (vitamins A, C, E, B-1, B-5, B-6, zinc, and selenium) can supplement DMSO. Bioflavonoids, such as pycnogenol, are also potent antioxidants.

* Vitamin C has been shown to help strengthen capillary walls.

* Iron supplementation is necessary for anemic individuals.

* Yellow Dock and Dandelion or liquid chlorophyll are a good source of iron.

Beneficial supplementation:

Vitamin A:
B Complex:
Folic Acid:
Vitamin C:
Vitamin D:
Vitamin K:

Bioflavonoids:
Calcium:
Iron:
Magnesium:
Zinc: 30 mg daily
Bromelain:
Herbs: Black Walnut, Comfrey, Dandelion, Horsetail, Kelp, Rose Hips, Slippery Elm, White Oak, and Yellow Dock.

How to avoid:

For those who are overweight, proper diet and weight loss are important. For those who are anemic, adequate iron intake is important.

Increase intake of foods high in vitamin C: citrus fruits and fruit juices, berries, cabbage, green vegetables and potatoes.

Avoid excessive intake of aspirin.

BURNS

Burns may be of three degrees; First degree burns: Cause redness and results in damage to the outer layer of skin only, such as sunburn, contact with hot object, hot water or steam.

Second degree burns: Cause redness, swelling, pain, blistering, and result in injury to skin beneath the surface of the skin. Second degree burns include deep sunburn, burns from hot liquids, gasoline and other substances.

Third degree burns: Cause destruction of all layers of the skin and underlying muscles. Burned area may be white or charred. There may be little or no pain because nerve endings have been destroyed. Third degree burns include prolonged contact with fire, hot substances or electrical burns.

What to do:

For first degree burns: Place burned area under cold, running water and apply cold water compress until pain subsides. Ice water will draw out heat and ease pain.

For second degree burns: Place burned area under cold water (not iced) or apply cold compresses such as a clean towel or wash cloth until pain subsides. Gently dry and cover burned area with a dry sterile bandage or clean cloth to prevent infection. Elevate burned arms or legs. Seek medical attention if necessary.

For third degree burns: Do not remove clothing that is stuck to burned area. Do not put ice or water on burns. Do not apply ointment, sprays or antiseptics.

Other suggestions:
     * Increase intake of fluids in treatment of burns.
     * Vitamin E can also alleviate pain and prevent blistering when applied immediately.
     * Aloe Vera can be used on first degree burns and after healing on second and third degree wounds to

prevent scarring.

* A diet high in protein helps aid in tissue repair.

* Intravenous vitamin C (30 to 100 grams) has been beneficial for individuals with third degree burns to maintain sufficient oxygen levels in the tissues and avoid the need for skin grafts.

* Do not apply butter or greasy ointment to burns. These are not sterile and can make subsequent treatment by a doctor more difficult.

* Essential Fatty Acids can help increase healing time.

Beneficial supplementation:

Vitamin A: 100,000 IU daily for a month for severe burns

B Complex: (extra B-12)

Vitamin C: 1,000 mg at least twice daily (1,000 mg hourly for severe burns)

Vitamin E: (externally and internally)

Multi-mineral:

Zinc: 50 mg

Protein:

EFA: 2-3 capsules three times daily

Herbs: Aloe Vera, Comfrey, Horsetail, and Slippery Elm.

How to avoid:

Never smoke in bed or when drowsy.

Set water heater thermostats or faucets so that water does not scald the skin.

Plan emergency exits to use in case of fire.

Apply suncreen with a SPF 15 or higher to all exposed areas of skin to avoid sunburn. **NOTE:** See section on skin cancer.

Supervise children and teach them fire safety as soon as possible.

CANCER

Most people are scared to death of cancer. But, while cancer is the among the top two causes of death today, the most common types of cancer are largely **preventable.** Chemical and environmental factors may be responsible for 90 percent of all cancers. Exposure to these factors is greatly are our own responsibility. Additional cancer risk factors which are more difficult to control include genetics, age, and to some extent, hormones and radiation.

Environmental and chemical factors include the following: sexual practices, use of alcohol, tobacco, many drugs and chemicals, presence of carcinogens and chemicals in food, stress (and how you deal with it), exercise, obesity, and finally, diet and nutrition.

While I will present a brief overview, I cannot possibly do this subject justice and therefore strongly recommend two excellent books; *Cancer and Nutrition* by Dr. Charles Simone, M.D. (Avery Publishing) and *The Cancer Industry* by Ralph Moss (Paragon House Publishing). These are outstanding books and well worth the small investment.

Cancer cells are abnormal cells which cannot fulfill their normal functions in the body. These cells multiply uncontrollably to form tumors which invade neighboring tissues causing problems. They rob normal cells of essential nutrients causing wasting. Cancer cells can also spread and progressively create havoc throughout the entire body. Symptoms depend on the type and location of the cancer.

Free radicals are largely responsible for the development of abnormalities and cellular damage. When free radicals damage the cell's genetic material, RNA and DNA, the cell mutates.

103

The key to fighting cancer is to prevent it.
Abnormal cells which are potentially cancerous are continually produced throughout the body. It is the responsibility of the white blood cells to rid the body of these abnormal cells before they can multiply and cause harm. But, continued exposure to carcinogenic substances such as tobacco, pesticide residues, and chemicals found in certain drugs, etc., weakens the immune system. If the body is maintained in good health standing, not abused or overwhelmed with chemicals in foods or drugs, stress, obesity, nutrient deficiencies, then the body can fight off cancerous cells, keeping them in check. Through diet and supplementation we can provide the immune system all it needs to keep us healthy.

Cancer-fighting phytochemicals are found in various foods like **Broccoli, Cauliflower,** and **Brussels Sprouts**. Such foods contain a host of disease-fighting, immune-promoting compounds which render carcinogens harmless.

Broccoli is also a good source of **vitamin C** (a powerful antioxidant which also stimulates T lymphocytes to produce interferon and reduces harm from nitrates), as are **tomatoes**, and many **berries** and **citrus fruits.**

Foods such as **Tomatoes, Pineapple, Strawberries,** and **Peppers** contain acids which also prevent formation of cancer causing agents in the body. Another acid found in **Strawberries, grapes** and **raspberries** also neutralizes carcinogens before they can cause damage.

Flavonoids, found in **all fruits and vegetables,** especially **citrus** and **berries,** keep cancer-causing hormones from latching onto cells.

Garlic and **Onions** contain sulfides that seem to protect against stomach cancer. They stimulate enzymes within cells which detoxify cancer-causing chemicals.

Peppers are loaded with special phytochemicals which keep certain carcinogens from binding to the genetic material in cells, where they can cause damage.

The health benefits of **beta carotene** are widely recognized. While **carrots** usually receive most of the glory for providing large amounts of this protective nutrient, beta carotene is also found in dark-green leafy vegetables like **Kale, Spinach, Broccoli,** and fruits like **Cantaloupe** and **Papaya.**

Antioxidants are renowned for the protection they offer us against oxygen damage and free radicals (damaged cells missing an electron). Free radicals are believed to be partially responsible for the effects of aging. Free radicals cannot be completely avoided as they are produced as a part of normal cellular function. Antioxidant nutrients donate one of their many electron to stabilize and neutralize the harmful effects of the free radicals. Without antioxidants, free radicals rob electrons from somewhere else, causing cells to weaken and become susceptible to damage.

Anthocyanidins, such as pycnogenols, found in many **berries** and **fruits**, are believed to be the <u>most potent form of antioxidants</u> available in nature.

Over a hundred different studies suggest that eating fruits and vegetables rich in vitamin C, beta carotene, anthocyanidins or taking an antioxidant supplement is linked to a reduced risk of virtually all cancers.

14 Easy Steps To Cancer Prevention:

1. Maintain ideal weight. Even if you are only 5 pounds overweight, lose it by decreasing the number of daily calories (eliminate all saturated fat) and exercise regularly. Keep active. Take the stairs instead of the elevator. Walk a few blocks instead of always taking the closest parking spot.

2. Eat a low-fat, low-cholesterol diet: Increase intake of vegetable protein sources such as beans, which are naturally low in fat and contain no saturated fat. Fish, especially those types rich in omega-3 fatty acids, is also good. Eat non-fat dairy products instead of the high fat ones. Avoid or eliminate red meat, especially processed meats, such as luncheon meats which contain nitrates. Avoid or eliminate fried foods. Limit oils and fats. Learn to enjoy the taste of foods without butter, sour cream, or other fatty condiments.

Animal fats increase bacteria in the colon which produce carcinogens. Animals fats slow down transit time (the time it takes to eliminate the waste products from the food consumed). The longer these carcinogens linger in the intestinal tract and colon, the more time they have to create trouble! Fiber increases transit time and helps carry fats out of the body.

3. Eat lots of fiber, at least 30 grams a day. The average consumption in the U.S. is probably less than 10 grams per day. Include fruits, vegetables and *whole* grains. For example, oatmeal is good, but *whole oats* or *steel-cut oats* are much better). Eat a variety of high fiber foods such as barley, millet, quinoa, amaranth, flax seed, lentils and beans.

Colon cancer is the second most common form of cancer. Red meat, cholesterol, animal fat and low fiber consumption, along with sedentary lifestyle, are the major contributors to colon cancer. Remember, animal products (meat and dairy) contain no fiber at all!

4. Eat lots of fruits and vegetables (especially cruciferous): Broccoli, cabbage, cauliflower, brussels sprouts, tomatoes, carrots, have all been shown to contain numerous anti-cancer phytochemicals.

5. Utilize nutritional and herbal supplements: Supplement your diet with vitamins, minerals, antioxidants and herbs in the proper dosages and combinations for your lifestyle.

6. Avoid Chemicals: Eliminate MSG, salt, nitrates, and food additives. Eat no barbecued, smoked, or pickled foods. Eat organically grown foods whenever possible.

7. Avoid caffeine: Coffee, tea, many soft drinks, chocolate and many other substances contain caffeine, a harsh stimulant and diuretic.

8. Avoid Tobacco: Do not smoke, chew, or inhale other people's smoke.

9. Avoid Alcohol: Consume only minimal amounts (one drink per week). Alcohol creates havoc on the liver, brain cells, and immune system.

10. Avoid Radiation: Have X-rays taken only when necessary. Use a sunscreen with an SPF of at least 15 when outdoors. (See the chapters on aging and skin cancer for more information on this subject.)

11. Maintain a healthy environment: Keep air, water, and work place clean. Regulate electromagnetic fields.

12. Avoid drugs: Avoid promiscuity, hormones, and any unnecessary drugs.

13. Avoid Stress: Exercise is a great way to relax. Meditation and prayer have shown to have a beneficial effect on the immune system and health.

14. Be familiar with what is normal for you. Everyone's body is different. Learn the 7 Early Warning Signs of Cancer:
*   Lump in breast.
*   Change in wart or mole.
*   Sore which will not heal.
*   Change in bowel or bladder habits.
*   Persistent cough or hoarseness.
*   Indigestion or trouble swallowing.
*   Unusual bleeding or discharge.

Find a physician whom you trust to monitor your ongoing health status through regular checkups. It is always better when a problem is detected early. Best, of course, is prevention through the 14 easy steps outlined above.

Beneficial supplementation:

B-Complex vitamins: (especially folic acid, riboflavin pyridoxine, pantothenic acid, and cyanocobalamin)
Antioxidant nutrients such as:
Vitamin A: (especially protects membranes in lungs, mouth and nasal passages) 50,000 IU
Beta carotene,
Vitamin C: (buffered, such as in the form of ascorbates) 5-40 grams daily
Vitamin E: Strengthens cell membranes against invasion of viruses and toxic chemicals. Up to 1200 IU daily
Pycnogenol: 100-300 mg.
Zinc: Boosts anti-cancer activity of the T cells. 100 mg
Selenium: Helps build gluthione perioxidase, an enzyme in all cells which acts as a powerful antioxidant. 100 mcg.
NAC (N-acetyl cysteine):
L-Methionine:
L-Glutathione:
SOD (superoxide dismutase):
Germanium: This anti-viral mineral boosts interferon production in the body. Among many other sources, it is found in aloe vera and exists in extremely high concentrations in the so called "healing waters" throughout the world.
Chromium picolinate: 400 mcg. daily
Sulfur:
Magnesium:
Molybdenum:
Phosphorus:
Lactobacillus acidolphilus: Especially protective against colon cancer
Potassium:
Amino Acids: Especially L-carnitine which improves fat utilization.
Flax seed: High in lignin fiber and Omega-3 fatty acids. Add 2 teaspoons freshly-ground seeds to

protein shakes, cereals, non-fat cottage cheese, non-fat yogurt, baked goods, etc.

Shark Liver Oil: Contains alkylglycerols which stimulate immunity through increased production of white blood cells. This oil has also shown to reduce incidence of injuries among individuals undergoing radiation therapy.

Evening Primrose Oil: An excellent source of Omega-3.

Herbs:
Alfalfa (high in fiber, saponins and trace minerals)
Astragalus (potent antioxidant)
Burdock root (anti-tumor activity)
Chaparral (anti-inflammatory, promotes healing)
Echinacea (immune booster)
Garlic and onion (immune boosters)
Ginkgo Biloba (powerful antioxidant)
Ginseng (stimulates healing and immunity)
Goldenseal (stimulates immunity)
Turmeric (anti-inflammatory, promotes healing)

Alternative Therapies:
The bottom line: *The body has the ability to heal itself.* A number of natural therapies are successfully utilized throughout the world, and have been for many years. But, most, if not all, are defamed unacceptable and ineffective by the established medical community in this country, largely for political reasons. Regardless of their potential value, most "natural methods" are "shunned." For those seeking additional information on alternative therapies I suggest contacting the following organizations:

Laetrile (Vitamin B-17) and Metabolic Therapy:
American Biologics Mexico S.A. Medical Center
180 Walnut Avenue
Chula Vista, CA 9201
(619) 429-8200
1-800-227-4458 (Outside California only)
1-800-227-4473 (Inside California only)

Burzynski and Antineoplastons:
Burzynski Research Institute
Outpatient Clinic
6221 Corporate Dilve
Houston, Texas 77036
(713) 777-8233

Research Institute
12707 Trinity Drive
Stafford, Texas 77477
(713) 240-5227

Hydrazine Sulfate:
Syracuse Cancer Research Institute, Inc.
Presidential Plaza
600 East Genesee Street
Syracuse, NY 13202
(315) 472-6616

Vitamin C:
Linus Pauling Institute of Science and Medicine
440 Page Mill Road
Palo Alto, CA 94306
(415) 327-4064

General Information:
People Against Cancer
PO Box 10 Otho
Iowa 50569
1-800-NO CANCER

CHOLESTEROL REDUCTION

Cholesterol is a fatty substances manufactured largely by the liver and intestines, but also by all cells in the body, for the production of the adrenal sex hormones, vitamin D, and bile salts. Cholesterol also has a vital role in nerve and brain function.

In food cholesterol is found in animal fat, not vegetable fats. Cholesterol is manufactured from dietary saturated fatty acids and refined carbohydrates. Foods high in cholesterol include egg yolks, cream, butter and fatty meats including organ meats.

Egg (1 medium)	274 mg.
Steak (8 oz.)	208 mg.
Lamb chops (6 oz.)	168 mg
Veal cutlet (6 oz.)	168 mg.
Hamburger (6 oz.)	162 mg.
Pork chops (6 oz.)	150 mg.
Ham (6 oz.)	150 mg.
Ice cream (1 cup)	59 mg.
Chocolate pudding (1 cup)	36 mg.
Whole milk (1 cup)	33 mg.
Ricotta (1/4 cup)	32 mg.
Cheddar cheese (1 oz.)	30 mg.
Mozzarella (1 oz.)	15 mg.
Butter (1 tsp.)	12 mg.
Mayonnaise (1 tbsp.)	9 mg.
Skim milk (1 cup)	4 mg.

High blood cholesterol levels increase your risk of heart attack and stroke. Here is why: Cholesterol is carried in the blood stream where some is deposited in the inner linings of the arteries. These fatty deposits buildup causing the artery walls to thicken and become less flexible. The artery narrows and restricts blood flow. Eventually the blood supply may be shut off completely. If the blockage is in an artery feeding the brain a stroke may result. If the blockage is in an artery which feeds the heart, a heart attack may occur.

There are different types of blood cholesterol levels which can be measured, for example, HDL (High Density Lipoprotein) and LDL (Low Density Lipoprotein) cholesterol levels. These are the two main types of cholesterol in the body.

HDL refers to the type of cholesterol returning through the blood stream back to the liver. This will then hopefully convert into bile salts when fat is eaten and be excreted with fiber. HDL is sometimes called "good cholesterol" because it is hopefully on its way out of the body.

LDL cholesterol travels through the bloodstream and delivers cholesterol to the tissues and glands that in turn use it to produce hormones, etc. LDL is sometimes called "bad cholesterol" because it may very easily get trapped in plaques and clogged arteries.

On the other hand, HDL cholesterol seems less likely to become so trapped. HDL ("good") helps clear LDL cholesterol from the bloodstream by transporting it to the liver where it gets broken down and excreted.

The HDL level may be as low as 30 or 40, or as high as 100 or 150. This number is compared to the total serum cholesterol to form a ratio. For example, if the total serum cholesterol is 250 and the HDL level is 100, the ratio would be 250 over 100 or 2.5 to 1. Generally, the lower the ratio, the better the health.

Total serum cholesterol levels checked alone without HDL and LDL levels, may be very deceiving. For example, if the total level is 200, it may look satisfactory to a physician. But, if the HDl level is only 20 milligrams, the ratio would be 10 to 1, which indicates higher than twice the average risk to experience a heart attack.

The amount of cholesterol that we absorb from the foods we eat is not 100 percent. Most people can absorb no more than 300-500 mg per day of cholesterol from foods. In fact, up to 80 percent of blood cholesterol comes from production in the liver, not from the cholesterol in the food we eat. Only 20 or 30 percent of the cholesterol in our blood comes preformed from cholesterol-containing foods we eat, no matter how much we eat.

Even if we ate absolutely no cholesterol, everyday the liver would still make up to 1,500 mg of cholesterol from fats and sugars. The components to make this cholesterol comes from foods we actually **should** cut down on eating: Saturated animal fats and simple sugars, including sucrose (white sugar), fructose, and corn syrup. The liver is an expert in converting sugars into cholesterol. On average, American's eat 150 lbs of white sugar per person a year which gives the liver a tremendous amount of raw material to turn into cholesterol.

What to do:

* Vitamin C helps increase HDL levels, lower LDL levels and lower triglyceride levels. It also dramatically reduces high elevations of blood cholesterol by activating the conversion of cholesterol into bile salts.

* Vitamin B complex, lost in the refining process of starches and essential in the metabolism of carbohydrates is known to help keep cholesterol from collecting.

* Vitamin E, also removed in the refining of grains and oils, helps dissolve clots, dilates blood vessels and conserves energy so the heart can work less. Vitamin E is also an antioxidant.

* Niacin, known to reduce cholesterol levels as much as 25 percent, is even more effective when used with oat bran.

* Lecithin, which contains choline, is essential for the proper use of fat and cholesterol in the body. Lecithin in the diet significantly lowers cholesterol levels.

* Essential Fatty Acids, found in flax seed oil, salmon, cod, and other cold water fish oils rich in Omega 3 decrease platelet adhesion, increase bleeding time, reduce blood cholesterol and increase HDL.

* Bran fiber also reduces blood cholesterol and triglycerides, increases HDL, and lowers LDL. Fiber also prevents cholesterol from recycling to the liver from the bowel, which signals a reduction of bile from the bowel back to the liver, which signals a reduction of cholesterol conversion to bile, causing a blood cholesterol increase.

* Avoid saturated animal fats and simple sugars, including sucrose (white sugar), fructose, and corn syrup. These are converted to cholesterol in the liver.

* Alfalfa is an excellant and effective supplement to aid in cholesterol reduction. Alfalfa is rich in saponins which provide a sort of sudsing action which prevents cholesterol and bile salts from being absorbed. Studies with alfalfa have demonstrated a 20 percent drop in total cholesterol. Ratios between high-density lipoproteins and low-density lipoproteins inproved by 40 percent. Alfafa also has demonstrated a beneficial effect on high blood pressure.

* Eating onion and garlic may help reduce heart disease. They both reduce the blood's tendency to clot. Raw onion and raw onion juice raises the levels of HDL. (Cooking reduces the beneficial chemical activity.) A clove or two of garlic can lower cholesterol and triglyceride levels in the blood.

* Eating apples (one to two daily) has shown to lower total cholesterol levels by approximately 10 percent. In addition, while LDL (bad) cholesterol decreased, the HDL (good) cholesterol increased.

* Lactobacillus acidophilus, cultured milk products, brewer's yeast, chromium, alfalfa, garlic, onion, and soy protein have all demonstrated ability to lower cholesterol.

* Physical activity and exercise are also important factors necessary to reduce elevated cholesterol levels, particularly HDL levels.

* Stress, caffeine, cigarettes, alcohol, and obesity are all factors which contribute to heart disease and should be avoided.

* Chelation therapy, or EDTA (Ethylene Diamine Tetraactetic Acid), is a nonsurgical alternative aimed at increasing blood flow. It involves a simple binding of a metal ion within a carrier molecule, which allows the transport of the metal ions through the body. This causes a change or balancing of other ion metals.

EDTA, a man-made amino acid, collects calcium in the blood stream (which otherwise binds cholesterol to artery walls) and toxic metals such as cadmium, mercury and lead. The kidneys remove EDTA and any calcium or metals bound to it, and flushes them out.

The body then readjusts and replaces the calcium in the blood by releasing calcium from other sources. This brings about gradual withdrawal of the calcium in the plaque of the arterials with a widening of the arterial lumen and relaxation of the arterial walls, resulting in better circulation. The plaque in the arteries becomes softer, and the vessels become stronger, more supple and better able to tolerate larger quantities of blood without raising the blood pressure.

The cholesterol is thought to be removed by two ways, either excreted or gobbled up by scavenger cells within the body.

Beneficial supplementation:

B Complex: 25-50 mg one to three times daily
B-6:
B-12:
Biotin:
Choline:
Folic Acid:
Inositol:
PABA:
Niacin: 3,000 mg daily
Pantothenic Acid:
Pangamic Acid:
Vitamin C: 3 grams daily
Vitamin D:
Vitamin E: 400 IU two to three times daily
Unsaturated Fatty Acids:
Bioflavonoids:
Kelp:
Lecithin:
Calcium:
Chromium: 600 mg daily
Magnesium: 300 mg to 2 grams daily
Potassium:
Selenium: 100 to 200 mcg daily. (Helps improve efficiency of vitamin E.)

Vanadium:
Zinc:
Fiber: such as brans, pectin,
Alfalfa: 2,000 mg 3 times daily
L-arginine:
L-carnitine: 1,500-3,000 mg daily
Herbs: Angelica, Black Cohosh, Hawthorn,
Hawthorn and Walnut combination, and
Mistletoe.

Beneficial foods: Alfalfa, apples, barley, beans
(pinto or navy), carrots, chili peppers, eggplant,
garlic, grapefruit, skim milk, oat bran, olive oil,
onions, seafood, seaweed, soybeans, spinach,
yams, and yogurt.

How to avoid:

Choose lean meat, fish, poultry, dried beans and peas
as protein sources.

Moderate or eliminate use of eggs and organ meats
such as liver and kidneys.

Use skim or low fat milk and dairy products.

Avoid hard cheeses, cream cheese and semisoft
cheeses. Stick to cottage cheese, ricotta, mozzarella (part
skim), and parmesan.

Eliminate use of saturated fats such as butter,
cream, shortenings, coconut oil, palm oil and foods made
with such products.

Choose oils which are high in polyunsaturated fats
such as olive, safflower or sunflower.

Avoid sausage, bacon and processed luncheon meats.

Trim fat off meats.

Bake, broil, and boil instead of frying.

Limit fatty salad dressings, gravies and sauces.

Moderate or eliminate consumption of refined
carbohydrates and sugar.

Read labels carefully to determine amounts and type
of fat in food.

116

COLD SORES

Cold sores or canker sores can be caused be allergies (foods such as coffee, tea, wheat germ, pork, turnips, cabbage, eggs, and milk), stress, and a virus, Herpes Simplex Type I. Canker sores have also been found among individuals who are deficient in iron, folic acid, and vitamin B-12.

What to do:

Following are several valuable and proven remedies:
* Make a paste with Golden Seal, Black Walnut, and Aloe Vera juice and put on infected area.
* Apply Myrrh in alcohol solution with a cotton swab.
* Apply an ice cube on the cold sore for 45 minutes. (Ancient but effective remedy.)
* Apply Vitamin E (28,000 IU) externally for 15 minutes three times daily.
* At first sign apply zinc, which is anti-viral, topically.

Beneficial supplementation:

Vitamin A:
B Complex:
Vitamin B-5 (pantothenic acid):
Vitamin B-12:
Folic Acid:
Vitamin C: 1,000 mg at least twice daily
Vitamin E: Internally and externally
Calcium:
Magnesium:
Iron:
Phosphorus:
Selenium:
Zinc: 50 mg daily and also topical
L-Lysine: 1,000-4,000 mg daily

Lactobacillus acidophilus: Three capsules three times daily

Herbs: Aloe Vera, Capsicum, Comfrey, Garlic, Golden Seal, White Oak Bark, and Myrrh (in alcohol solution applied topically).

COMMON COLD

The common cold is a general inflammation of the mucous membranes of the respiratory passages caused by a variety of viruses. Because there are so many different types of viruses, it is difficult to develop a cure or cold vaccine. Colds are highly contagious and are spread through hand to hand contact. This is sometimes referred to as "The Devil's Circle."

Symptoms include nose and throat irritations, sneezing, runny or stuffy nose, watery eyes, headache, fever, chills, muscle aches and temporary loss of smell and taste.

On average most people suffer from two or three colds per year. Most colds last about seven days.

What to do:

* At first sign of cold symptoms increase vitamin C intake to bowel tolerance level. Bowel tolerance level, according to Dr. Linus Pauling, is the level of vitamin C in the body which causes diarrhea. Once you achieve this level reduce intake. This level can vary greatly from person to person (8 to 100 grams per day), depending on their state of health at the time.

* Increase intake of foods which contain vitamin C, including citrus fruits, fruit juices, berries, cabbage, and green vegetables.

* It is important to replace lost vitamins and minerals due to the stress of a viral infection. The most prevalent are vitamin C, B Complex and zinc. Zinc loss contributes to the loss of taste and smell commonly associated with colds and flu.

* Zinc is known to revive the key gland of the immune system, the thymus. Research shows that as little as 15 mg can improve immune function, by restoring immune function in even the elderly. Zinc also provides antibacterial/antiviral properties in the mouth so it may

119

be beneficial to suck zinc lozenges or gargle with mouthwash which contains zinc. **NOTE:** Do not use high amounts of zinc for more than a week because it may upset your system.

* Echinacea is effective against viral and bacterial attacks, not by killing these organisms but by supporting the body's natural defense system. In some situations it stimulates the body's own antibiotic chemicals to become more active or to increase. Echinacea is very beneficial in the prevention and treatment of colds and flu, as well as upper respiratory infections, tonsillitis, and mouth and throat infections. The effectiveness of echinacea increases when used in conjunction with vitamin C and garlic

* L-lysine is beneficial for viral infections.

* Beta carotene (vitamin A) protects the lungs,

* Hot herbal teas, especially those containing peppermint, are effective to help open nasal passageways.

* Increase liquid intake, especially hot.

* It also may help to inhale steam to warm the nasal passageways. Germs can not thrive in an environment above 103 degrees fahrenheit. For this reason many authorities recommend that aspirin should be avoided. Aspirin lowers the body's temperature which is the natural immune response of the body. A heightened body temperature makes the white blood cells more mobile and more effective in killing germs. In addition, interferon, a protein produced by the body to fight off the virus, works less efficiently when the fever is brought down.

* Do not smoke and avoid those who smoke.

* If possible, stay home and in bed to reduce strain on yourself and avoid spreading the virus to others.

* If cold symptoms persist longer than 14 days or if your temperature is above 103 degrees F., see your doctor.

Beneficial supplementation:

Vitamin A: (Beta carotene is preferred because high dosages can be safely utilized)
B Complex:

Vitamin C: 1,000 mg every three hours for first three or four days, 500-1,000 mg daily. Higher dosages are also recommended to bowel tolerance.

Vitamin D:

Vitamin E:

Unsaturated Fatty Acids:

Bioflavonoids:

Calcium:

Zinc: 30 mg two to four times daily

Acidophilus:

Protein:

L-Lysine:

Water: eight or more glasses per day

Herbs: Alfalfa or Peppermint teas, Raspberry tea combinations, Lemon-Lime Aloe Vera drink, Echinacea, Fenugreek, Garlic, Ginger (settles stomach), Golden Seal, Kelp, Marshmallow, Rose Hips, and Slippery Elm (for coughs and throat).

How to avoid:

Maintain indoor humidity of 45 percent or above because the membranes of the nose, throat and lungs are less vulnerable to irritation and viral infection. Use a gauge to check humidity levels and if necessary, turn on a steam vaporizer to increase the level.

Hand to hand contact spreads more colds than does sneezing, coughing or kissing. You can also catch a cold from a door handle, telephone receiver, sink, etc. because a cold virus can remain volatile upon such surfaces 72 hours after touched by an infected individual. Hygiene is extremely important. Wash your hands as often as possible and avoid touching your face as much as possible.

Maintain adequate sleep, diet, exercise, and levels of stress. Other factors which lower our resistance to virus infection include overexposure to cold, allergic reactions, and inhalation of irritating dust or gas.

Did You Know...

Milk retains it nutrients better in fiberboard cartons than in clear plastic? When exposed to fluorescent light, low-fat or skim milk loses 90 percent of its vitamin A in 24 hours.

CONSTIPATION

Constipation is characterized by difficulty in passing your stool. Commonly this is due to a diet lacking bulk (fiber) and water, high in animal products, especially dairy, and a lack of exercise. Constipation can also result from the use of antacids and certain medications such as codeine.

Severe chronic constipation is a common disorder among the elderly. This is commonly due to sedentary lifestyle and poor diet.

Constipation is often caused by travel (due to changes in water, diet and daily activities), pregnancy, hypothyroid function, aluminum toxicity, and stress.

What to do:

* Increase intake of water, fiber and increase exercise.

* Helpful foods include: Garlic, flax seed, fruit, especially apples, papaya, pineapple, prunes, and figs.

* Take 60 mg folic acid each day.

* Supplement Lactobacillus acidophilus or eat yogurt which contains Lactobacillus acidophilus daily. **NOTE:** Avoid any yogurt which contains sugar, corn syrup or other artificial sweeteners.

* Harsh laxatives can rob the body of nutrients, as well as cause rebound constipation and laxative dependency. Laxative abuse can damage the internal wall of the colon and destroy intestinal muscle tone. Avoid harsh laxatives such as senna, castor oil, phenolphthalein, magnesium hydroxide, magnesium sulfite, and sodium sulfite.

* Increase exercise if lifestyle is sedentary.

* Drink fig, prune, or raisin tea.

Beneficial supplementation:

Vitamin A: 25,000 IU
B Complex:
Vitamin B-1: 100 mg
Choline: 500 mg
Inositol: 500 mg
Folic acid: 60 mg daily
Vitamin C: 1,000 mg
Vitamin D:
Vitamin E:
Unsaturated fatty acids:
Acidophilus:
Water: At least 8 glasses daily
Fiber: Ground flax seed, apple pectin, bran,
  psyllium seeds or husks, etc.
Herbs: Cascara Sagrada, Comfrey, Garlic,
  Psyllium, Slippery Elm, and Triphala (Chinese
  colon tonic).

How to avoid:

Maintain a diet high in fiber (whole grains, fruits, vegetables, and unrefined bran), drink eight glasses of water daily, and get adequate amounts of exercise.

Avoid eating a diet high in dairy products because they tend to be constipating among many individuals.

Maintain adequate levels of exercise.

Avoid aluminum containing products such as antiperspirants and beverages from aluminum cans.

DANDRUFF

Dandruff is a mild inflammation of the scalp causing flaking. These flakes are often highly visible on the hair and can fall off onto the shoulders.

Dandruff may be caused by nutritional deficiencies such as vitamins B-6, B-12, F (essential fatty acids), and selenium. In addition, inefficient carbohydrate metabolism has been associated with dandruff. Sugar is often the trigger.

Dandruff which is more serious is called seborrheic dermatitis. It is caused by overactive seborrheic glands which are irritated by emotional trauma, illness, or hormonal imbalance.

What to do:

* Shampoos containing selenium are effective in controlling dandruff flakes. Shampoo hair and scalp at least once a week. Leave in shampoo for at least five minutes before rinsing. If you shampoo daily do not use a selenium shampoo every time you wash your hair.

* Peanut oil and lemon are effective in controlling dandruff. Rub warm peanut oil into the scalp. Then apply fresh lemon juice. Leave on for a few minutes and shampoo.

* Try rubbing vinegar into the scalp.

Beneficial supplementation:

Vitamin B-6:
Vitamin B-12:
Vitamin C:
Vitamin E:
Vitamin F (essential fatty acids): Flax seed oil, fish
   oil, etc.
Selenium:

Zinc:
Evening Primrose Oil:
Lecithin:
Antioxidants:
Herbs: Burdock and Yucca.

DIABETES

Diabetes is a metabolic disorder characterized by decreased ability or complete inability of the body to utilize carbohydrates (glucose). Diabetics have an insufficient production of the hormone insulin which is essential for the conversion of glucose to energy. Therefore, in the diabetic, glucose cannot be converted to energy and instead is accumulated in the blood resulting in symptoms that range from mental confusion to coma.

Diabetes is a chronic degenerative disease, meaning all vital organs and tissues are affected by the condition in a negative manner. Diabetes can often lead to additional complications such as atherosclerosis, loss of sight, kidney disease, gangrene, coma and premature death.

Symptoms of diabetes include extreme thirst, frequent urination, sugar in urine, increased appetite, loss of weight, fatigue, muscle cramps, impaired vision, itching, and slow healing wounds.

The following factors are associated with the development of diabetes: High intake of simple carbohydrates (especially sugar), nutritional deficiencies, excess intake of saturated fat, pregnancy, surgery, physical or emotional stress, adrenal exhaustion, heredity, and obesity.

Types of diabetes include:

Type I: Insulin-dependent diabetes mellitus, also called juvenile-onset or congenital diabetes. Type I diabetes starts in children, tends to be unstable and is hard to control.

Type II: Non-insulin-dependent diabetes mellitus, also called adult-onset diabetes. The disease usually begins after the age of 40, but can occur at any age. 60-90 percent of individuals are overweight. Individuals are not dependent upon insulin although many may use it for control of symptoms.

What to do:

The possibility of cure by natural means depends on the severity of the case and the length of insulin dependency.

While congenital or juvenile-onset diabetes can never be corrected completely through diet alone and will always require insulin, proper diet does help moderate the condition.

Mild cases of adult-onset diabetes are easy to control. If insulin is used for prolonged periods, the pancreas may be suppressed to the degree that it has literally ceased to function. The body can become dependant upon exogenous insulin and reduce its own insulin production.

* A diet high in unrefined carbohydrates is the most beneficial for diabetics of all types. The diet should consist of no simple carbohydrates and no sugar, and no refined carbohydrates.

* Fats consumed should be vegetarian and unsaturated.

* No red meat should be consumed and chicken and fish should be restricted to several times per week. Vegetarian protein sources are recommended such as whole grains, nuts (almonds, cashews, peanuts, etc.), seeds (pumpkin, sesame, sunflower,) etc. soybeans, black beans, kidney beans, navy beans, pinto beans, etc.

* Some diabetics may need to avoid fruit and fruit juices, depending on their individual condition.

* About 75 percent of the diet should be composed of raw foods.

* Meals should be small and eaten five to six times a day.

* Some foods have a natural insulin-like action in the body and should be included in the diet in high quantities. These include:

Brewer's yeast
Brussels sprouts
Buckwheat
Cucumbers
Fiber (wheat bran, oat bran, guar gum)
Garlic
Green beans
Jerusalem artichokes
Oatmeal or oat flour products
Raw vegetables
Soybeans and tofu
Spirulina
Wheat germ

* Maintain regular levels of exercise.
* Inositol is often used to prevent and treat neuropathy which is commonly associated with diabetes.

Suggested supplementation:

Vitamin A: 10,000 IU
Vitamin B-1: 10 mg
Vitamin B-2: 10 mg
Vitamin B-5 (pantothenic acid):
Vitamin B-12: 25 mcg
Vitamin C: 4,000+ mg
Vitamin E: 400-1,000 IU
Bioflavonoids:
Calcium:
Chromium picolinate: 200 mcg
Magnesium: 500 mg
Manganese:
Potassium: 300 mg
Zinc: 100-150 mg
Lecithin: 3 or more tbsp daily
Raw pancreas tablets:
Raw adrenal tablets:

Spirulina:

Herbs: Alfalfa, Burdock, Garlic, Goldenseal (acts an insulin), Red Clover, Uva Ursi, Watercress, and Yellow Dock.

How to avoid:

A proper diet (high in complex carbohydrates, low in fat, low in red meat, minimal to no refined, simple carbohydrates, etc.) in most cases will prevent diabetes from occurring, particularly Type-II adult-onset diabetes.

DIARRHEA

Diarrhea, passing of loose watery stools, can be caused by parasites, food poisoning, colitis, stress, viruses, chemicals, allergies, and food allergies, such as milk.

Diarrhea can exist alone or as a symptom of other diseases. Diarrhea is commonly accompanied by increased thirst, abdominal cramps and bloating, intestinal rumbling and loss of appetite.

Because of the rapid movement of food through the digestive tract, individuals with diarrhea do not properly utilize and absorb nutrients.

What to do:

* To avoid dehydration, drink lots of water.
* Yogurt contains friendly bacteria which helps normalize bowel functions. Yogurt also has an antibiotic effect, especially against E. Coli, the main cause of traveler's diarrhea.
* Carob powder, which is high in pectin, helps stop diarrhea.
* Fiber such as bran helps normalize bowel function.

NOTE: A diet high in fiber or bran may decrease the body's ability to absorb minerals such as iron and calcium. To avoid complications you may wish to eat foods containing calcium and iron at different times from when you eat large amounts of fiber.

* To replace lost nutrients, supplement your diet with the nutrients listed below, especially the B-Complex vitamins, vitamin C, sodium, potassium, magnesium, which are bound closely to water which is lost when you have diarrhea. Your diet should be rich in protein, carbohydrates, essential fatty acids, and other vitamins and minerals as well.
* If diarrhea lasts longer than two days, seek medical attention. Prolonged diarrhea can cause severe dehydration.

Beneficial supplementation:

Vitamin A:
B-Complex:
Vitamin C: 1,000-3,000 gm
Potassium:
Sodium:
Calcium: 2,000 mg
Magnesium: 500 mg
Zinc:
Protein:
Acidophilus:
Herbs: Alfalfa, Glucomannan, Raspberry (tea), and
Slippery Elm.

How to avoid:

Maintain a healthy diet, proper exercise and sufficient water.

Avoid eating contaminated food (see section on food poisoning).

DIETING AND OBESITY

Obesity is a national health problem. It is estimated that 60 million Americans are above their ideal weight.

An individual becomes overweight when more calories are consumed than the body can burn off by activities. The excess calories are stored in the body as fat. The more calories taken in above what is burned off, the more fat accumulates. Each 3,500 excess calories equals one pound of body fat.

Obesity exposes you to numerous risks and even premature death. Overweight individuals are more prone to kidney disease, diabetes, high blood pressure, liver disorders and arthritis.

What to do:

The only way to lose weight is to eat less (consume less calories) and exercise more. Nutritionally balanced and low calorie meals combined with a suitable exercise program can keep excess weight off permanently.

Reduction of calorie intake alone without exercise is not likely to produce desired weight loss results. When less calories are taken than the body is accustomed to, the body's rate of metabolism slows down. Exercise increases the body's rate of metabolism therefore compensating for the difference.

Avoid crash dieting because it can be dangerous. Sudden weight loss can damage the heart, gastrointestinal tract and metabolism.

Tips:

* Eat three balanced meals every day. Avoid snacking and do not skip meals.
* Tighten your belt before meals.
* Drink a glass of water before you eat.
* Have a cup of low calorie soup and eat a salad (with

low calorie dressing) 10 or 15 minutes before your
meal.
* Eat more fiber. Fruits, vegetables, whole grains and
beans add bulk to the diet and make one feel full.
* Cut down on simple carbohydrates and empty
calories such as sugar and sweets, and alcohol.
* Cut down on fats. Avoid fried foods, fatty meats,
and skin from chicken.
* Eat slowly. Try to eat smaller bites and put your
fork down in between bites.
* Try putting meals on smaller plates.
* Use herbs and spices to flavor food instead of high
calorie dressings and toppings.
* Chinese Ephedra (Ma Huang) has thermogenic or
fat burning effects on the body. Ephedra
stimulates the Alpha-II-adrenalin modulated
pathways found on various tissue in the body.
When these sites are stimulated the metabolic
activity of the tissues increases. There are high
amounts of Alpha-II receptors on the tissues of the
body known to produce heat (which is why the
term thermogenic is used). Chinese Ephedra also
acts as an appetite suppressant.
* Growth hormone releasers, such as the amino acids
arginine and ornithine, may be beneficial to help
burn fat and build muscle. To be the most
effective, they should be taken on an empty
stomach before exercise or before you retire at
night .

When you feel the urge to snack or binge:
* Put on some of the clothes you would like to wear
but are too tight.
* Fill up on water.
* Brush teeth and tongue.
* Fiber taken with water, for example, Glucomannan,
guar gum or bran, can give one a feeling of
fullness.
* DL-Phenylalanine can be taken to suppress
appetite.
* If you cannot resist the urge eat only low calorie

fresh fruits or vegetables (cauliflower, cucumbers, mushrooms, celery, carrots, apples, oranges, etc.).
* Avoid artificial sweeteners, for example, those found in diet drinks. Artificial sweeteners are many times sweeter than sugar so they cause a craving for sweets.
In addition, artificial sweeteners may fool the body into thinking it has ingested sugar. As a result, your body releases extra insulin that can lead to weight gain.

Beneficial supplementation:

B Complex: (extra B-2, B-6, B-12, choline, folic acid, inositol, and pantothenic acid)
Vitamin C: 1,000 mg
Vitamin E: 600 IU
Calcium: 500-1,000 mg
Magnesium: 250-1,000 mg
Phosphorus:
Zinc:
Protein:
DL-Phenylalanine: 100 to 300 mg
Lecithin:
Essential fatty acids:
Fiber:
GHR (Arginine and Ornithine): 2-4 times daily preferably on an empty stomach
Raw pancreas:
Raw pituitary:
Raw thyroid:
Herbs: Bladderwrack (fucus), Kelp, Garlic, Glucomannan, and Ma Huang.

How to avoid:

Read food labels for sugar, sodium and fat content. The order the ingredients are listed is according to quantity. For example if sugar is the first ingredient listed, that means there is more sugar in the product than anything else.

Do not overeat.

Eat balanced meals consisting largely of complex carbohydrates including: whole grains, fruit, and vegetables; protein including beans, sprouted beans, sprouted seeds, nuts in moderation, low-fat yogurt, poached eggs, chicken, turkey and fish; and cold pressed unsaturated fats.

Exercise on a regular basis.

Use stairs or walk whenever possible.

DIGESTIVE DISORDERS

Digestive disorders include gastritis, heartburn, and indigestion, which are symptoms of abnormal digestion. These are characterized by acute or chronic abdominal discomfort, pain, irritation, bloating or gas, often accompanied by general malaise, headache, nausea, and sometimes vomiting.

Contributing factors include:
Improper diet-refined carbohydrate and sugar, overeating, insufficient chewing of foods, hurried meals, snacking, strong spices, salt, coffee, tea, alcohol, carbonated beverages, acid-forming foods, food additives, preservatives, and colorings, food allergies, etc.

Digestive enzyme activity, constipation, cigarettes, candida albicans overgrowth, bacterial overgrowth, drugs including aspirin, stress, lack of exercise, heavy metals, obesity, pregnancy, etc.

What to do:

First and foremost, diet changes are necessary.
* Eliminate consumption of refined carbohydrates, especially sugar. Refined carbohydrates cause a rapid secretion of gastric acid. This acid is normally buffered by the protein content of a food substance, but bran and fiber are removed in the refining process. Green vegetables are the best alkaline element for maintaining proper pH balance.

* Eliminate excessively large meals. When the stomach is overloaded, the digestive enzymes cannot "keep up with the work load" and food which is not completely digested is passed on to the lower small intestine. The result is indigestion, fermentation, and gas. Eating too often can create the same problem. Wait at least 1 1/2 hours after a fruit meal, 2 to 2 1/2 hours after a vegetable meal and 3 to 4 hours after a combined meal

with proteins, carbohydrates, and fat.

* Slow down and chew your food. Chewing of food is part of the digestion process. Digestive enzymes in the mouth break food down into smaller particles for more adequate digestion in the stomach.

* Acute cases may require fasting with water with a twist of lemon, dilute apple juice, carrot juice, carrot and cabbage juice or Slippery Elm tea. This may be followed by a mono diet regimen such as apple mono diet, carrot mono diet, or brown rice mono diet.

Beneficial supplementation:

Vitamin A: 10,000-25,000 IU daily
B Complex: 25-50 mg one to two times daily
Folic Acid:
Vitamin C:
Vitamin E: 400 IU two times daily
Bromelain
Charcoal tablets:
Pancreatic digestive enzymes:
Aloe Vera Juice: 2 ounces three times daily
Fiber:
Hydrochloric Acid: (if hypo-acid)
Kelp:
Lactobacillus Acidophilus:
Lemon Juice:
Papaya enzyme:
Pepsin:
Sodium Alginate:
Herbs: Angelica, Anise, Chamomile, Comfrey, Calamus Root tea, Dandelion, Fennel, Garlic, Ginger Root, Goldenseal, Papaya or Aloe Vera with meals, Peppermint, and Slippery Elm.

How to avoid:

Do not eat under stress.
Slow down and chew your food thoroughly.
Avoid refined carbohydrates and sugar.

DRY SKIN

Dry skin is a term to describe rough, scaly, and flaky skin, usually on areas below the neck, that is dry to the touch and less flexible or elastic than normal skin.

Dry skin is usually more common as winter approaches when the temperature drops and relative humidity decreases. This causes the skin to lose a large amount of water which leads to dry skin, scaling and occasional itching. Artificial heating, harsh soaps, and soaking too long in too hot baths can aggravate the condition.

In the summer months, sunbathing and air conditioning can contribute to problems with dry skin.

Dry skin can result from a deficiency of vitamins A, C, B Complex, or unsaturated fatty acids. Because the oils of the skin are largely unsaturated, the unsaturated oils are needed for moist skin.

What to do:

* Make sure you are getting adequate source of Vitamin A, such as provided by sweet potatoes, carrots, liver, etc., which can help dry skin.

* Apply Na-PCA, the skin's natural moisturizer whose production decreases as we grow older.

* Take one or two tablespoons of Cod Liver Oil (containing vitamins A, D and essential fatty acids) every morning on an empty stomach.

* Flax seed oil, which contains high amounts of essential fatty acids, has been reported to make skin soft, smooth and supple.

* After bathing or showering, apply a light oil, such as sesame, to areas of the body susceptible to dryness to seal in moisture. Do not put the oil directly into the bath water because the oil will cling to the skin and water cannot be absorbed through the skin.

Beneficial supplementation:

Vitamin A: 25,000 IU daily
B Complex: (extra B-2, B-6, biotin, and niacin)
Vitamin C: 1,000 mg daily
Vitamin D: 800 IU
Vitamin E:
Silicon:
Selenium:
Zinc:
Essential Fatty Acids: (Flax seed oil, Cod liver oil, Lecithin, etc.)
Water
Herbs: Alfalfa and Aloe Vera.

How to avoid:

Increase the relative humidity in your home to at least 40 percent.

When you shower or bathe, do not use extremely hot water or harsh soaps.

Avoid excessive sunbathing, cold temperatures, and strong winds.

Some experts suggest that eating acidic foods (orange juice, tomatoes, etc) is drying to the skin and therefore these foods should be avoided.

Drink at least eight glasses of water every day.

ENERGY

To obtain optimal energy levels or stamina it is necessary for the entire body to be in good health. It may be necessary to take measures to improve digestion and circulation, to cleanse the colon, to nourish the glands and organs (especially the lungs and heart) and to strengthen the nerves.

If the body is weak it functions poorly, resulting in sluggishness, lack of motivation, etc.

Under-nutrition produces deficiencies of critical nutrients, particularly the B Vitamins (especially the blood-forming nutrients: Folic acid, vitamins B-6 and B-12). These help to stimulate the body's synthesis of blood cells which carry oxygen to the tissues in the body and give rise to the production of energy.

Lack of energy could also be a result of a deficiency in the mineral family: Particularly iron, zinc, and chromium. These are also very important for the maintenance of proper energy levels.

There is a range of conditions that may give a person a feeling of lack of energy. Research shows that most of these are due to nutrient insufficiencies.

Energy levels are also dependant on adequate oxygen intake. You can increase your oxygen intake by doing deep breathing exercises.

Beneficial supplementation:

High potency multivitamin with chelated minerals:
Stress formulas (B Complex):
Vitamin B-6:
Vitamin B-12:
Folic Acid:
Chromium:
Iron:
Zinc:

Wheat germ oil (also called Octocosonal):
    NOTE: Allow four to five weeks to feel a difference.
Lecithin:
CoQ10:
Green Oats:
Bee pollen:
Herbs: Fo-Ti, Ginseng, Gotu-Kola,

How to avoid:

Avoid the following: Sugar, refined carbohydrates, caffeine, tobacco, alcohol, tea, coffee, soft drinks, processed and refined foods.

FATIGUE

Fatigue or lack of energy is probably one of the most common complaints heard in a doctor's office. Fatigue is a feeling of physical and mental weariness which can be caused by a variety of conditions, such as anemia, physical exertion, hypoglycemia, nutrient deficiencies (Vitamins C, D, B-Complex, folic acid, magnesium, potassium, copper, iron, and zinc) shallow breathing, medications, weight loss, obesity, boredom or emotional tension, stress, allergies, glandular imbalances, or almost any disease process. Fatigue is commonly accompanied by headaches, backache, irritability, and indigestion.

What to do:

One needs to find the cause of the fatigue and then treat it. Supplementation can be very beneficial if deficiencies are present. For example, iron poor blood cannot adequately carry oxygen throughout the body which usually results in fatigue, and a diet poor in potassium causes muscular weakness, irritability, and a tired feeling.

* If you are athletic and exercise regularly, make sure you eat enough foods which are rich in potassium or take a potassium supplement. Potassium helps cool muscles after exertion. Foods high in potassium include: apricots, broccoli, lima beans, peaches, dates, figs, and seafood.

* American Ginseng combined with Red Deer Antler (equal parts) is known as the most powerful energy-memory tonic for individuals of all ages.

* Adequate rest and a well balanced diet can prevent fatigue. If you are overweight, reducing weight to normal is necessary.

* Deep breathing can increase oxygen intake.

Beneficial supplementation:

Vitamin A: 25,000 IU daily
B Complex: 50 mg two to three times daily
Folic Acid:
Vitamin C: 1,000 mg three times daily or more
Vitamin D:
Chromium: (In the case of hypoglycemia especially)
Iron: 25-50 mg daily
Magnesium: 400-500 mg daily
Manganese:
Potassium:
Fiber:
Brewer's Yeast:
Bee Pollen:
Glandulars:
Kelp:
Spirulina:
Herbs: Cayenne, Ginseng, (American Ginseng and
Red Deer Antler combination) and Gotu Kola, and
Oats.

How to avoid:

Eat well-balanced meals and especially, do not skip breakfast.

Exercise more. Exercise increases your rate of metabolism and also helps relieve stress.

Sleep more. If you often become drowsy during the day, get an extra hour of sleep at night. In addition, it is important to maintain adequate sleep conditions. Avoid sleeping on a saggy mattress.

Work at your peak. Schedule tough jobs for the time of day you feel most energetic.

Take breaks. During work it helps to stop, stretch, walk, or relax.

Maintain good posture. This promotes greater lung expansion, which brings more oxygen into the brain, increasing alertness and decreasing fatigue.

Do deep breathing exercises.

Avoid sugar, refined carbohydrates and all artificial stimulants including coffee, caffeine, drugs, etc.

Make sure that you have adequate privacy. Lack of privacy contributes to stress and fatigue. Noise can also contribute to stress and trigger fatigue.

Did You Know...

Where the most germs are in your house? The most popular places for germs are in the kitchens and bathrooms. The most germs are in the sinks and bathtubs, U tubes, dishcloths, cleaning cloths, facecloths, and bathmats. Toilets are actually relatively germ free.

FLATULENCE

Flatulence (intestinal gas) is the most common digestive disturbance. Flatulence is abnormal amounts of gas passing upward or downward, with or without intestinal discomfort.

In infants, flatulence is commonly termed colic. It is accompanied by abdominal pain, distension, insomnia, fretfulness and hysteria.

Flatulence is caused by swallowed air and gases liberated by putrefactive bacteria that are living on undigested food. Excessive swallowing of air can occur while eating or drinking, eating too fast, or eating when anxious or upset. Eating too much food overwhelms the digestive enzymes. Undigested food becomes a breeding ground for putrefactive bacteria which form gas.

Milk products can also cause flatulence in cases of lactase insufficiency. Other foods which can cause flatulence are beans, cucumbers, cabbage, apples, whole grains, fried foods, concentrated sugar from dried fruits.

The most common cause of infant colic in the totally breast fed infant is the mother's diet. An inappropriate diet of fried foods, junk food, and refined foods is the usual cause. Any food may cause the infant distress, but the most common foods are cabbage, onion, garlic, wheat, yeast, brussels sprouts, and broccoli.

What to do:

* Efficient digestion depends on hydrochloric acid, bile, and other digestive secretions and enzymes.
* Fermented foods such as yogurt and buttermilk aid in the digestion of high fiber foods by increasing friendly bacteria in the colon.
* Carminative herbs stimulate digestion by increasing gastric juices, decreasing the amount of putrefactive bacteria and stimulating intestinal motility. These include garlic, anise, fennel, and caraway.

147

* Exercise stimulates intestinal movement and breaks down large gas bubbles.

* Charcoal tablets which absorb gases in the digestive tract are very beneficial.

* Fennel is a natural remedy for gas and stomach acid. This herb can be sprinkled on food to prevent stomach gas.

* Use Goldenseal as a bowel tonic. Use 25 drops in water three times per day.

* Drink hot water with lemon juice.

Suggested Supplementation:

B Complex:
Vitamin B-5 (Pantothenic acid):
Digestive enzymes:
Hydrochloric acid:
Bile:
Acidophilus:
Chlorophyll:
Charcoal tablets: One to two per hour in acute cases
Herbs: Alfalfa, Anise, Blessed Thistle, Capsicum (cayenne), Caraway, Fennel, Garlic, Goldenseal, Peppermint, and Wild Yam.

How to avoid:

Avoid hurried meals and inadequate chewing.

Avoid eating under stress.

Avoid eating foods which are known to cause flatulence. Never eat fried foods, hydrogenated fats, sugar, refined carbohydrates or other junk food.

Avoid eating fruits and vegetables at the same meal.

Avoid a diet containing sugar, refined carbohydrates, excess meat and low in fiber content.

Avoid eating between meals.

Avoid drinking large quantities of liquids with meals.

FLU

The term "flu" can actually refer to two different conditions. Stomach flu (gastroenteritis) is the inflammation of the lining of the stomach. This inflammation can have a variety of causes including food poisoning, certain viruses, alcohol intoxication, sensitivity to drugs, and allergies.

Flu also can be short for influenza, which is acute viral infection of the respiratory tract. Influenza is highly contagious and easily spread by coughing and sneezing

Gastroenteritis is characterized by diarrhea, vomiting, possible fever, chills, and abdominal cramps that vary in severity, head and body aches, possible chest pain and cough, and extreme fatigue. Recovery is usually within one or two days.

Influenza is characterized by chills, high fever, sore throat, headache, abdominal pain, hoarseness, cough, enlarged lymph nodes, aching of the back and limbs, and frequent vomiting and diarrhea. Serious complications can occur, for example, pneumonia, sinus and ear infections.

What to do:

* If possible, stay in bed.
* Drink plenty of liquids.
* Do not smoke. Cigarette smoking weakens resistance and lung power.
* Supplement vitamin C to bowel tolerance.
* Garlic, which contains allicin, is antibiotic which destroys harmful bacteria in the body without interfering with the body's natural bacteria.

Beneficial supplementation:

Vitamin A:
B Complex:
Vitamin B-1: 50-200 mg
Vitamin B-2: 10 mg
Vitamin B-6: 50-100 mg
Niacin: 50-100 mg
Pantothenic acid: 25-300 mg
Vitamin C: 3,000-15,000 mg
Potassium:
Protein:
Herbs: Garlic and Symfre.

FOOD POISONING

Food poisoning results from eating foods infected by poisons or by bacteria containing toxins. Symptoms for food poisoning include nausea, vomiting, diarrhea, and abdominal cramps. If symptoms persist for more than 24 hours, seek medical attention. Dehydration and serious complications can occur with food poisoning.

Common bacteria which cause food poisoning:

Salmonella: There are 1,700 types of salmonella bacteria which are commonly found in raw meat, poultry, milk, and eggs. Flies, insects and pets can carry this bacteria. Salmonella is the leading cause of food poisoning deaths in America. Symptoms develop within 8 to 36 hours of eating contaminated foods. Symptoms may include severe headache, diarrhea, cramps, nausea and vomiting.

Staphylocci: This is the most common bacteria causing food poisoning which develops in meat, poultry, egg products, custards, cream-filled pastries, potato salad and many other foods. Staphylocci is most often caused by food standing too long at room temperature. Symptoms (vomiting, cramps, and diarrhea) develop within one to eight hours after eating contaminated food.

Escherichia Coli: This bacteria is the main cause of traveler's diarrhea. It is often transported in the water supply because of sewage contamination. Symptoms (mild to severe diarrhea) occur within 8 to 44 hours after ingestion.

Botulism: Food may be toxic due to toxins produced by germs before the food is eaten. Botulism is usually fatal. Its growth occurs in under-processed, non-acid canned foods and multiplies profusely in the absence of oxygen. Boiling will destroy the toxin. Symptoms include weakness, headache, nausea, vomiting, sometimes diarrhea and abdominal distress, constipation and retention of food in the stomach. After 12 to 14 hours, double vision, and difficulty talking and swallowing will occur. If these symptoms occur, seek medical attention immediately. If medically untreated, cardiac and respiratory failure can occur and death will occur in three to seven days. Over 50 percent of those poisoned die.

What to do:

* If symptoms persist for more than 24 hours, seek medical attention. If double vision or difficulty talking or swallowing occur, seek medical attention immediately.
* Replace lost fluids, minerals and water soluble vitamins with supplements when vomiting subsides.
* Lactobacillus acidophilus has proven to be an excellent preventative for traveler's diarrhea.

How to avoid:

Food poisoning is commonly the result of improper handling of food or improper hygiene. Always make sure hands and fingernails are thoroughly clean before handling food.
* Keep hot foods hot and cold foods cold. Hot foods should be kept at 140 degrees or hotter. Cold foods should be stored at less than 45 degrees. Foods kept between these temperature are prone to rapid bacterial growth.
* Cook meats, especially pork and poultry, thoroughly in order to kill harmful bacteria. Heat kills bacteria.
* Guard against the growth of harmful bacteria by immediately refrigerating leftovers or foods cooked for later use. Do not allow them to cool to room temperature first.
* Keep perishable foods, especially chopped and processed meats, custards, pastries and dairy products, in the refrigerator to avoid bacterial contamination.
* Destroy cans that bulge or canned contents that bubble out when the can is opened. Avoid unusual colored food. If a food looks bad, never taste for spoilage. Even a tiny amount of bacteria can be dangerous.

* Avoid eating meat from livestock fed antibiotics because it may contain drug-resistant bacteria. When eaten, this bacteria can lead to serious illnesses including salmonella-especially if you recently took antibiotics yourself.

* Before cooking raw beef and poultry, rinse them under cold running water. If you chop the pieces, wash the utensils and cutting board with hot soapy water before they touch other food.

* Supplemental hydrochloric acid can help prevent some forms of food poisoning.

* Pet turtles are thought to carry salmonella, so avoid contact with them or make sure you wash thoroughly after handling them.

Did you Know...

Licorice may be hazardous to your health? A chemical in licorice which resembles steroid hormones can have the same ill effects if you eat too much (about two pounds).

Licorice and licorice flavoring also contains glycyrrhizic acid which can cause hypertension and fatigue. **NOTE:** Ex-smokers and alcoholics are particularly susceptible to licorice's harmful effects.

FOOT PROBLEMS

Over eighty percent of us suffer from aching feet. It is the third most common medical complaint. Following are a few common food ailments:

An **ingrown toenail** is inflammation caused by a toenail whose top edge is pressed into the skin of the toe. Nearly all cases are caused by confining shoes, improper hygiene and nail cutting. Treatment includes wearing wider shoes, proper trimming of nail, and surgery to narrow the nail.

A **bunion** is abnormal swelling of the joint at the base of the big toe. It is caused by swelling of the bursa (cushion that allows the tendon to move over the bones of the joint), usually the result of long-term irritation and pressure from poorly fitted shoes, pronation, supination or imbalance of the foot.

A **callus** is a common, usually painless, thickening of the skin at any location of the foot of pressure or friction. It can be caused by underlying bone problems which cause excess irritation, where shoes repeatedly rub and dead skin cells accumulate.

A **corn** is a cone-shaped horny mass of thickened skin on the toes resulting from long-term friction and pressure. The conical shape of the corn presses down on the skin beneath, making it thin and tender. There are two types of corns. The hard corn is most often found on the outside of the little toe or the upper surfaces of the other toes. The soft corn is found in between toes and kept soft by moisture. Treatment includes relief from pressure and surgical or chemical removal.

Hammertoe is a toe permanently bent at the middle joint, giving a claw-like appearance. They are produced by a muscle imbalance which cause the end of the joints to bend down, while the closer joints bend up. It is most common in the second toe although it may be present in more than one.

Plantar Fascitis or Heel Spurs are a chronic inflammation of the plantar fascia, a ligament-like structure that passes from the heel to the forefoot. The inflammation is caused by the fascia partially pulling away from the heel. A bony spur, which may or may not cause pain, is caused by excessive heel rotation, excessive heel pounding, or longitudinal arch weakness.

Tendonitis is a swelling condition of the tendons in the foot. It usually results from a strain. Treatment usually includes rest and support.

Foot Odor: Another plague of modern living is feet which sweat, smell and offend when shoes come off. This is because the feet need to perspire in order to eliminate accumulations of fluids and toxins. The feet being at the bottom of the body, naturally receive some of the heavier fluids and minerals. Since the feet are also at the distal end of venial system, circulation tends to be weak. Sweating is therefore a necessary process.

What to do:

* In general, it is important to restore normal circulation to the feet by massage, spinal manipulation or possibly liver cleansing.

* Soak foot in warm salt water. Carefully remove dead granulated tissue.

* Wear comfortable shoes that fit.

* Avoid high heels and cowboy boots.

* The best natural method of soothing and softening these common foot ailments, is with frequent applications of Castor Oil. The oil can be applied any time during the day, but is most efficient when applied on the afflicted area just before going to bed. Rub the Castor Oil on liberally, and then put on a cotton, or wool sock. Do this nightly for three weeks. Then as often as needed, or desired.

* For an ingrown toenail, apply castor oil pack or slip a piece of cotton soaked in castor oil under the edge of the ingrown toenail to keep it pointing upward and out.

* For heel spurs, vitamin B-6 is beneficial.

156

For Sweaty Feet:
1. Soak one to three teaspoons of White Willow Bark (Salix alba) in one cup of cold water for two to five hours. Then bring this mixture to a boil. Add this to a tub of hot water, and soak feet for 15 to 20 minutes.
2. Add one pound of Chamomile Flowers (Matricaria Chammomilla) to five quarts of cold water. Bring to boil, cover and steep for 10 minutes. Strain and add to footbath. Soak feet for 15 to 20 minutes.
3. Boil one pint dried English Walnut leaves (Juglans regia) in one and one-half quarts of water for 45 minutes. Add to hot footbath, and soak for 15 to 20 minutes. This is also good for gout.

Herbal Foot Powders:
1. Powdered Hemlock Spruce (Tsuga Canadensis) is effective in reducing foot bacteria which causes odor. It is also shown to be beneficial in cases where ulcers are present. Simply sprinkle powder into socks and shoes.
2. Powdered Black Walnut Leaf is also a good foot powder, with excellent anti-fungal properties.

How to avoid:

To avoid corns, callouses, bunions, ingrown toenails, etc., wear comfortable, low healed shoes that fit properly.

To avoid sweaty smelly feet, avoid shoes and socks which are made from unnatural materials and are treated with chemicals. Polyester and other synthetics increase the body temperature, which increases perspiration. This use of chemicals and synthetic materials in our shoes and socks cause further problems which compounds this situation. The sweat combines with many of these chemicals, and result in fungus-like growths, and skin irritations of the feet.

Go without shoes as often as possible.

Properly fitting orthotic devices may also be beneficial

in both prevention and treatment of foot problems, especially fallen arches.

GALLSTONES

Gallstones are hardened, stone-like masses formed when deposits of cholesterol or calcium combine with bile. Bile is secreted by the liver to emulsify fats so they can be digested. Most of the bile manufactured is stored in the gallbladder until the small intestine calls for it when fats have been ingested. However, some bile travels directly from the liver to the small intestine. Gallstones may form in the passage between the liver and gallbladder, between the liver and intestines, or in the gall bladder itself.

Symptoms of gallstones include nausea, vomiting, and severe right abdominal pain that may radiate to the right shoulder or back. Symptoms will commonly occur a few hours after eating a heavy meal of fatty or fried foods. If a gallstone totally obstructs one of the bile passages, jaundice, dark urine, clay colored stools, and itching of the skin may also occur.

The following persons have an increased risk of developing gallstones: Diabetics, obese individuals and overweight individuals who frequently lose weight and then gain it back, individuals with high cholesterol levels, elderly people, and females, especially those who have had two or more children.

A diet high in cholesterol and deficient in vitamin C has been shown to cause the development of gallstones. Vitamin C is necessary for the conversion of cholesterol into bile acids.

What to do:

* Take adequate amounts of vitamins A, B Complex and E.
* B Complex vitamins increase the body's production of lecithin and also stimulate the emptying of the gall bladder.
* Lecithin and bran reduce cholesterol levels.
* Chamomile tea, dandelion tea and dandelion greens

159

each help clear obstruction.

* Supplement olive oil plus lemon.
* Drink one quart of apple juice daily for five days. On the sixth day, skip your evening meal and at 6 p.m. take a tablespoon of epsom salts with water. Repeat in two hours. At 10 p.m. make a cocktail of four ounces of olive oil and four ounces of fresh squeezed lemon juice. Shake vigorously and drink. In the morning you will pass green stones, but will not feel a thing.
* Drink lots of grapefruit juice.
* The combination of choline, inositol and methionine make good lipotropics to stimulate bile.
* Yellow Dock also helps bile production.

Beneficial supplementation:

Vitamin A: 10,000-25,000 IU daily
B Complex: 24-50 mg two to three times daily
Vitamin C: 1,000-2,000 mg two to six times daily
Vitamin D:
Vitamin E: 400 IU one to three times daily
Vitamin K:
Lecithin: one to two capsules three or four times daily
Olive oil: Include in diet daily
EPA (Eicosapentenoic acid): 5-10 grams daily
Bran:
Herbs: Chamomile, Dandelion, and Yellow Dock.

How to avoid:

Reduce the amount of saturated fat and excess carbohydrates in the diet.
Eat adequate quantities of bran and lecithin.
Avoid long intervals between meals.
Maintain adequate levels of vitamin C.
Maintain adequate levels of exercise.
Avoid birth control pills.
Avoid stress.
Drink eight glasses of water daily.

GOUT

Gout is a condition of faulty protein processing which results in high levels of uric acid in the system. Excess acid is converted to sodium urate crystals that settle into joints and other tissues. It is very painful. The great toe is a common site for buildup of urate crystals. Gout can also occur in the heel, hand, fingers, ear, or any joint in the body. The condition can result in red, painful swelling of a joint, along with chills and fever.

Gout affects men more often than women and victims are usually over age 40. Approximately 10-20 percent of individuals with gout have an inherited form of gout.

Gout is commonly associated with excess meat consumption (particularly organ meats), excess refined carbohydrates and sugar (increases uric acid levels), overindulgence in alcoholic beverages, excess coffee, lack of fresh fruits and vegetables, acidosis, obesity, lack of exercise, stress (executive syndrome, adrenal exhaustion), and lead poisoning.

What to do:

* Non-citrus alkaline fasting (vegetable juice, non-citrus juice, red cherry juice) is an excellent method for eliminating excess uric acid from the system and re-establishing equilibrium

* Red cherries (canned, fresh, frozen or concentrate) relieves the pain of gout by neutralizing uric acid.

* Drink lots of water-three quarts a day.

* Eat a diet high in complex carbohydrates and low in fat and protein. Decrease or end consumption of meat, especially organ meats.

* Avoid alcoholic beverages.

* For acute attack, use 5-15 drops Colchicum tincture daily.

161

Beneficial supplementation:

Vitamin A: 25,000 IU
B Complex (extra B-5):
Vitamin C: 5,000 mg daily
Vitamin E: 400-800 IU daily
Calcium:
Magnesium:
Potassium:
Bioflavonoids
Herbs: Burdock Root, Colchicum (tincture), Guggula, Celery, and White Bryony (tincture - for pain made worse by motion).

How to avoid:

Drink adequate amounts of water daily.

Avoid excess consumption of meat, protein, refined carbohydrates, and alcohol.

GRAY HAIR

Graying hair can indicate a deficiency of nutrients such as vitamin E, copper, folic acid, pantothenic acid, and or PABA, in other parts of the body.

What to do:

* A return of normal hair color has been accomplished by supplements of copper, folic acid, pantothenic acid, and or PABA.

* Take 800 IU of vitamin E every day. Foods rich in vitamin E include dark green vegetables, fruits and rice.

* Have a hair analysis done to find out exactly which minerals or trace minerals you are deficient in.

* Combine equal parts of black strap molasses, apple cider vinegar, and raw honey in a glass jar and mix thoroughly. Once daily mix 2-3 teaspoons of the combination into hot water and drink.

Beneficial supplementation:

B Complex:
Folic Acid: 5 mg daily
Pantothenic Acid: 300 mg daily
PABA: 300 mg daily
Magnesium:
Zinc:
Sulfur
Copper:
Herbs: Mulberry Fruit, Privet, Eclipta, in general, yin tonics.

GUM DISEASE

Gum disease, also called periodontal disease or pyorrhea, is the inflammation and infectious condition of the structures that support the teeth. It is a progressive disorder caused by the bacteria found in plaque.

Plaque is an invisible bacterial film which forms on the teeth made up of material found in saliva and other particles. It is constantly forming in the mouth everyday. Everyone produces plaque, even those who care for their teeth. It is necessary to remove plaque on a daily basis. If allowed to build up under the gum line, these bacteria thrive and multiply. Along the roots of the teeth, plaque will become calcified, often called tartar, which can only be removed by your dentist. Eventually, this can cause tooth decay, tooth loss, and periodontal disease.

Smoking, a poorly fitted filling, dental bridgework or an abnormality where the teeth meet, all encourage progression of bacteria growth.

Periodontal disease is the major cause of tooth loss among adults. It is estimated by age 60, nearly 40 percent of the adult population needs false teeth as a result. The condition usually affects people over age 30 and becomes more prevalent with age, possibly due to the cumulative effects of bacteria. Without proper maintenance, even young people may experience some forms of periodontal disease.

After the common cold, gum disease is the most common infectious ailment in this country. According to the American Academy of Periodontology, "Of the 125 million American adults who still have their teeth, 100 million are now infected and an estimated 32 million have an advanced case."

There are two common types of periodontal disease, gingivitis and periodontitis, each caused by different type of bacteria found in plaque. Unfortunately, both diseases often go unnoticed by the individual since they are usually painless. The sooner one receives treatment the

165

better and of course prevention is always the best treatment.

Gingivitis is a superficial inflammation of the gums. It usually begins with swollen, red gums that may bleed during brushing. Later, bad breath or a bad taste in the mouth may be present. Gingivitis usually does not result in tooth loss.

Periodontitis is caused by more harmful bacteria that affect not only the gums but the supporting bone, which can eventually result in bone loss. The bacteria colonize in the gum crevices around teeth and to the tooth root surfaces. The bacteria emits toxins that inflame the gum tissue and the gums will begin to pull away from the teeth. The inflammation can spread all the way into the bone underneath and cause serious damage by deterioration. As the infection advances, "pockets" can form between teeth and the supporting tissues. Eventually the teeth will loosen and fall out.

Traditional methods of correction include surgery, reconstruction and regeneration of damaged tissue and bone. Non-surgical procedures may be attempted if disease conditions are treated early enough.

What to do:

* Dentists agree that the best treatment for tooth and gum problems is prevention. Daily removal of plaque and regular visits to your dentist will help keep your teeth and gums healthy.

* Brush and floss after every meal.

* Brush your teeth with baking soda or tooth powders containing baking soda.

* Rinse your mouth daily with a diluted hydrogen peroxide solution.

* Rinse your tooth brush in hydrogen peroxide.

* Vitamin C, zinc and calcium have shown to be effective.

* Rub chlorella into the gum line.

* Vitamin C has been shown to help protect the gums against infection. In addition to supplements, there are

some mouth washes available which contain vitamin C. Because zinc is antibacterial in the mouth, it also may be helpful to use a mouthwash which contains zinc.

Beneficial supplementation:

Vitamin A: 25,000 IU daily
B Complex: 25-50 mg one to two times daily
Folic acid:
Vitamin C: 1,000-2,000 mg three to four times daily
Bioflavonoids:
Vitamin E: (chewable) 400 IU daily, plus local application to gums.
Calcium:
Zinc: 15-25 mg one to two times daily
Trace minerals:
Cod liver oil:
Lactobacillus acidophilus:
Chlorella:
Herbs: Cayenne, Coneflower, Goldenseal, and Myrrh.

How to avoid:

Careful brushing and flossing at least two or three times a day is the best defense.

Have your teeth cleaned regularly by a professional. They can get to areas where brushing and flossing cannot.

Avoid a high-phosphorus and refined diet which is the major cause of tooth and gum disease. Eat a diet high in raw fruits, raw and lightly cooked vegetables, nuts, fermented dairy products and whole refined grains. Avoid excess meat, soda, candy, refined cereals and overcooked foods.

If you cannot brush your teeth after eating, chew on foods like carrots or celery which help rid the teeth of bacteria and make your mouth cleaner.

A calcium deficiency can weaken the bones which house the teeth and make the body more susceptible to infections. Calcium has been shown to be a key factor in the prevention and treatment of gum disease. Foods high in calcium include low-fat milk, green leafy vegetables, legumes, salmon and lowfat yogurt.

Hydrogen peroxide can be used to kill bacteria and prevent gum disease. Dip toothbrush in hydrogen peroxide and then hydrogen peroxide and salt. Smear this mixture along the gum line into all crevices between the gums and teeth. Rinse thoroughly. This kills bacteria and foams it away. According to the International Dental Foundation, this is an effective method to help prevent gum disease.

If a dentist informs you that you have periodontal disease and that he wishes to do treatment, you may wish to get a second opinion. Many times unnecessary treatments are prescribed.

HAIR CARE

Nutritional deficiencies can be one of the major causes of hair problems. Optimal blood circulation is dependant upon nutrition. A well-balanced diet is important to maintaining healthy hair, although hereditary graying and balding cannot be completely prevented by nutritional means.

Because hair is primarily protein (98 percent), a deficiency in any of the amino acids can result in color or texture changes or hair loss. If the deficiency is corrected, the hair will return to its normal condition.

A vitamin A deficiency can cause hair to become dull, dry, lifeless, and eventually fall out. However, an excess of vitamin A may cause similar problems.

Stress, or deficiency of the B vitamins (especially biotin, pantothenic acid, inositol, choline, PABA, and folic acid), or zinc, copper, magnesium, sulfur can trigger hair loss. In addition, an underactive thyroid, excess copper, and intoxication by heavy metals, such as mercury, lead and cadmium, also cause hair loss.

Stress can also damage your hair because tension restricts blood vessels in the scalp reducing its supply of oxygen and nutrients. Hair loss can be the result. Excessive hair loss, usually in patches, is known as Alopecia Areata. This usually is a temporary condition, but may result in total hair loss.

What to do:

A hair analysis may reveal which nutrients you are deficient in so proper supplementation can be made.

Treatment for alopecia areata includes B-vitamin complex, adrenal glandulars, gotu kola, and calming nervines such as valerian root, hops, chamomile, passion flower, etc. It is also important that one has an adequate intake of protein.

Warm sesame oil, castor oil and Kotu Kola massaged into the scalp may help stop hair from falling out.

169

Beneficial supplementation:

Vitamin A:
B Complex:
Vitamin B-6:
Biotin:
Folic Acid:
Inositol:
Choline:
PABA:
Pantothenic Acid:
Vitamin C:
Copper:
Iodine:
Magnesium:
Silica:
Sulfur:
Zinc:
Protein:
Herbs: Burdock, Chamomile, Comfrey, Horsetail,
   Jojoba, Nettle, Oat Straw, Peach, Sage, Gotu Kola
   with Eclipta together promote hair growth and
   Rosemary helps prevent hair from falling out.
Nervines: Valerian Root, Hops, Passion Flower, Goto
   Kola, Skullcap.

How to avoid:

Eat a well-balanced diet with lots of whole grains, nuts, seeds, fresh fruits and vegetables.

Maintain a diet adequate in protein.

Avoid exposure to the sun and wind. Wear a hat or scarf for protection. Wear a cap to protect your hair from chlorine when swimming. Shampoo hair immediately after swimming.

Maintain good hygiene with a mild shampoo.

Get regular trims. Trimming the hair makes it look fuller and healthier. This is because the older hair on the ends is more prone to splitting.

Never brush your hair when it is wet. Carefully use a

wide toothed comb or pick.

Use the proper type of brush on your hair. The best hairbrush bristles come from boars. Their uneven surface cleans better than smooth nylon. Black bristles are good for thick heavy hair. White bristles are better for fine or thinning hair.

Keep brushes and combs clean-they irritate the scalp and inhibit hair growth.

Remove split ends by cutting at least a quarter inch from your hair.

Hot oil treatments, mayonnaise, eggs, and yogurt have been used to combat frizzies and dry hair.

Avoid using hair products containing alcohol, which is drying to hair.

To brighten all shades of dull hair try chamomile extract.

Note: To remove gum or tar from hair, rub with vegetable oil, then wash with soap and water.

Did you Know...

If you add zinc to your diet to make sure to get enough vitamin A?

HEADACHE

Headache, or pain or ache in any portion of the head, is a symptom rather than a disease itself.

Headaches can be caused by stress, heavy metal toxicity, insomnia, depression, constipation, indigestion, sinusitis, head injury, air pollution, hunger, hypoglycemia, poor circulation and poor respiration. Additional causes include allergies to MSG, chocolate, caffeine and caffeine withdrawal, wheat, sulfites, dairy products, vinegar, poor dietary habits (sugar and refined carbohydrates, junk food, etc.), alcohol, toxins or fumes, liver disorders, menstrual disorders, anemia, high blood pressure, head injury, and eye strain.

Tyramine-containing foods (red wine, sherry, champagne, beer, aged cheese, chicken liver, citrus, pickled herring, chocolate, avocados, bananas, plums) can initiate an attack because they seem to cause vasoconstriction of the blood vessels in the scalp resulting in a reduced blood supply.

Sodium nitrate containing foods (hot dogs, bacon and other cured meats) can cause headaches.

Birth control pills and estrogen supplements can cause headaches as well as monosodium glutamate (MSG) which is commonly added to Chinese food.

There are several types of headaches including:
Sick headaches (from undigested food in the stomach, stress or menstrual disorders).

Bilious headache (from indigestion, overeating, lack of exercise) are experienced by dull pain in forehead and throbbing temples.

Nervous headache (from tension, mental strain, and worry) are usually made worse by bright lights or noises of any kind.

Sinus headaches (from allergies, hayfever, etc. from inflamed mucous membranes of the nose)- are often brought on by changes in the weather, onset of menstruation, or a head cold.

Migraine headaches are recurrent attacks of headaches often combined with visual and gastrointestinal disturbances. The pain is usually confined to one side of head or eye.

Repeated headaches may be a symptom of a serious disorder and therefore deserves medical attention.

What to do:

Treatment for headache depends on the underlying cause.

* Avoid sugar which can make headaches worsen.

* Colon cleansing may be helpful for bilious headaches.

* For a nervous headache, it may be helpful to lie down where it is quiet and massage neck muscles. Heat from a heating pad or a hot tub also helps.

* Soaking your hands in hot water can relieve nervous or migraine headaches. Fill a sink with water as hot as you can stand it. Place both hands in the hot water up to your wrists for 30 minutes. The heat of the water expands blood vessels in your hands causing increased blood flow. This draws blood away from bloated arteries in the head which cause the pain. The hot water also stimulates nerve endings in your hands which send relaxation signals to your brain and the hot water takes concentration away from your pain and directs it elsewhere.

* If headache is caused from a drop in blood sugar or hunger, eat something, preferably complex carbohydrates or protein.

* Apply pressure to pressure points. One is located at the second joint of the thumb. Use the thumb and index finger on the other hand to rub the joint vigorously. Use oil or hand lotion to lessen friction when massaging. Repeat the process switching thumbs. If headache is severe 10 minutes of vigorous massaging on each thumb may be required.

Another pressure sensitive area is located in the palm

area. Press your thumb of one hand and press the palm of another. Press as firmly as you can and massage gently. The palm contains nerve endings. Pressure on nerve endings can relieve persistent headaches.

The third area is located near the eyebrows centering above each eye. Using the knuckles of each of your thumbs press firmly for several minutes until pain of headache subsides.

The last pressure point is located in the triangle of flesh between the thumb and index finger. With your other hand squeeze this area with your thumb and index pinched together. Concentrate on the most sensitive area.

* Drink a cupful of peppermint, catnip, red sage or spearmint tea.
* Relax and get some fresh air.

Beneficial supplementation:

Vitamin A:
B Complex: (extra niacin, B-15, and pangamic acid)
Vitamin C: (with bioflavonoids) four grams
Vitamin E:
Calcium: 500 mg
Magnesium:
Zinc:
Herbs: Chamomile, Feverfew, Hops, Peppermint plus Catnip (tea for headaches of stomach origin), Red Sage, Skullcap, Spearmint (tea), White Willow, and Wood Betony.

How to avoid:

Avoid known causes of headaches such as caffeine, tyramine, sodium nitrate, monosodium glutamate and oral contraceptives.

Maintain a regular sleeping schedule.

Magnesium supplements have been shown to reduce frequency and severity of migraine headaches. A magnesium deficiency increases one's sensitivity to noise, light and other stimuli.

175

Feverfew, when taken regularly helps prevent migraine headaches.

HEARTBURN

Heartburn is a symptom of abnormal digestion. Heartburn discomfort occurs when acidic digestive juices and partially digested food back up into the esophagus (passageway between the mouth and stomach). This irritates sensitive tissues and causes "heartburn" discomfort.

An excess of fat, alcohol, and acidic foods such as coffee, citrus and tomatoes can contribute to heartburn. Eating too fast, when emotionally upset or exhausted can trigger heartburn.

What to do:

* Standing or sitting up straight will force acid and partially digested food back into the stomach.

* Drinking milk after eating can sometimes combat stomach acid and bring relief.

* Antacids containing sodium bicarbonate may be helpful to neutralize excess acid but should not be overused. Used on a regular basis, they disturb the body's acid/alkaline balance, creating a condition of alkalosis. Sustained alkalosis with a substantial intake of calcium in the form of milk or calcium-containing antacids creates milk-alkali syndrome, causing irreversible kidney damage.

* Antacids, by neutralizing all the acid in the stomach, also prevent efficient digestion and thus interfere with nutrient absorption.

* Chewable papaya tablets (which contain bromelain) after meals can be helpful.

Beneficial supplementation:

Vitamin A:
B complex:
Vitamin C:

Digestive enzymes: papaya (bromelain)
Pancreatic enzymes:
Acidophilus:
Herbs: Aloe Vera, Burnet, Gentian, and Peppermint.

How to avoid:

Avoid eating chocolate, peppermint, onions, garlic, cabbage and also avoid mixing these foods with alcohol.

Avoid fatty foods (especially butter, cream sauces, gravies, salad dressings, etc.).

Eat more protein foods.

When eating sit up straight and do not wear tight clothes.

Avoid eating rapidly and when upset or exhausted.

Stop smoking.

Lose abdominal weight (pressure on the lower esophagus).

HEMORRHOIDS

Hemorrhoids are dilated veins around the anus and rectum. They may be either internal or external.

Poor eating habits (refined foods, lack of fiber, etc.) are largely responsible for hemorrhoids. This type of diet tends to cause constipation which causes the pressure inside the colon to increase. Hemorrhoids can also be due to strain on the abdominal muscles due to factors such as heavy or improper lifting, pregnancy, overweight, or sedentary lifestyle.

Symptoms of hemorrhoids include swollen veins which frequently become irritated and bleed. Hemorrhoids also cause itching and burning.

Prevention of hemorrhoids is much easier than their cure.

What to do:

* Increase your intake of dietary fiber to about 20 grams per day. Eat high fiber foods, a daily salad and fresh fruits and vegetables.

* Avoid commercial laxatives which irritate the lining of the colon.

* Warm water soaks (sitz baths) can help relieve discomfort and keep the area clean.

* Alternate hot and cold therapy.

* After bowel movements, pat yourself clean with a damp cloth. Avoid tissue paper.

* Bioflavonoids, especially rutin, strengthen the capillaries.

* Vitamin E can prevent and dissolve blood clots.

* Hemorrhoids can be relieved by aloe vera gel, which also stimulates healing.

* Avoid lifting heavy objects.

* Moderate exercise has a generally beneficial effect on colonic function. However, strenuous exercise, such as weight lifting, can aggravate hemorrhoids.

Beneficial supplementation:

Vitamin A: 10,000 IU twice daily
B Complex: 25-50 mg one to three times daily
Vitamin B-6: 25 mg three times daily
Bioflavonoids:
Vitamin C: 1,000 to 2,000 mg two to three times daily
Vitamin E: 400 IU three times daily
Blackstrap molasses:
Fiber: (such as bran) One to two tablespoons with
   meals
Herbs: Stone Root (capsule and suppository), and
   Goldenseal (suppository).

How to avoid:

Eat bulky foods such as grain, leafy vegetables, and
fruits to help regulate bowel movements.
Drink plenty of liquids every day.
Never postpone a bowel movement. When nature
calls, answer as soon as possible.
Maintain moderate levels of exercise. Strenuous
exercise and heavy lifting can aggravate hemorrhoids.

HEPATITIS

Hepatitis is an inflammation of the liver due to infection or toxic substances. Infectious agents include viruses, bacteria, and parasites. Toxic agents include antibiotics, drugs, industrial solvents, anesthetics, carbon tetrachloride, and others.

Infectious hepatitis is contracted through blood, feces, contaminated food, water and shellfish.

Hepatitis begins with flu-like symptoms of fever, weakness, drowsiness, abdominal discomfort, and headache, possibly accompanied by jaundice. Soon extreme fatigue and loss of appetite occur. The liver will be tender and enlarged. The liver is unable to eliminate poisons allowing them to build up in the system; and it cannot store and process certain nutrients that are vital for the body.

What to do:

* A high-protein diet which is primarily lacto-vegetarian is recommended: Yeast, wheat germ, egg yolk, lowfat yogurt, acidophilus lowfat milk, tofu, soybeans and spirulina. The diet should also contain high chlorophyll foods such as raw and cooked green vegetables.
* Vitamin C injections (25-50 grams sodium ascorbate per day) may be necessary with calcium gluconate (1 gram per 10 grams of vitamin C).
* Consume absolutely no alcohol or saturated fats.
* Coffee (regular brewed, organic if possible) enemas assist in toxin removal of the liver. Do at least once daily.

Suggested Supplementation:

Vitamin A: 10,000-25,000 IU emulsified two to four
   times daily.
Folic acid: 5 mg three times daily

B Complex:
Vitamin B-12:
Vitamin C: 1,000 mg hourly in acute cases.
  Intravenously: 25-50 grams sodium ascorbate per day with calcium gluconate (1 gram per 10 grams of vitamin C).
Vitamin D:
Vitamin E: 400-1200 IU daily
Essential fatty acids:
Lecithin:
Raw Liver tablets:
Chlorophyll:
Spirulina: One tsp three to four times daily
Beet Juice:
Carrot Juice:
Herbs: Celandine (tincture: 1 to 10 drops three to four times daily), Culver's Root (tincture: 10 to 60 drops three to four times daily), Fringe Tree (tincture: 5 to 30 drops three to four times daily), Gymnema Sylvestre, and Oregon Grape Root.

How to avoid:

Improper diet will leave the liver more susceptible to infection by clogging it with unnecessary chemicals or toxins. A healthy system is better able to resist such invasions. Most cases of hepatitis occur when resistance to disease is low.

Sanitation and good hygiene is important to avoid infectious cases of hepatitis.

HIATAL HERNIA

This occurs when a portion of the stomach protrudes above the diaphragm-the muscular wall separating the chest and abdominal cavity. This results in a loss of function of the valve at the bottom of the esophagus allowing stomach acid to back up into the esophagus producing heartburn - usually in the area underneath the breast bone. The pain most often occurs at night when in a reclined position. Experts estimate that about 40-50 percent of the U.S. population suffers a hiatal hernia.

What to do:

* Elevate the head of the bed six to eight inches by placing blocks under the front legs of the bed.
* Standing or sitting up straight will force acid and partially digested food back into the stomach.
* Drinking milk after eating can sometimes combat stomach acid and bring relief.
* Antacids containing sodium bicarbonate may be helpful to neutralize excess acid but should not be overused. Used on a regular basis, they disturb the body's acid/alkaline balance, creating a condition of alkalosis. Sustained alkalosis with a substantial intake of calcium in the form of milk or calcium-containing antacids creates milk-alkali syndrome, causing irreversible kidney damage.
* Antacids, by neutralizing all the acid in the stomach, also prevent efficient digestion and thus interfere with nutrient absorption.
* Chewable papaya tablets (which contain bromelain) after meals can be helpful.

How to avoid:

Avoid foods such as coffee, citrus fruit, highly spiced and seasoned foods, and chocolate.

Avoid eating or drinking for several hours before going to bed.

Avoid tight fitting clothing around the waist.

Bending should be done with the knees, not the waist, to avoid abdominal pressure.

Eat a high fiber diet. (In countries where the population maintain a high fiber diet, such as Africa, hiatal hernia are unknown.)

HICCUPS

Hiccups are a involuntary contraction of the diaphragm. The noise is due to air being sucked in and suddenly stopped by tightened vocal cords.

Hiccups are caused by overeating or over drinking, indigestion, nervousness, exercising too soon after eating and faulty swallowing of food.

Usually hiccups only last for short periods of time, while there are cases where they have lasted for weeks or even years. Fortunately, most cases are easily relieved.

What to do:

* A high carbon monoxide level in the blood is known to inhibit most cases of hiccups. Therefore holding the breath and deep breaths, and re-breathing into a paper bag are the most commonly used techniques.
* Other commonly used methods include:
* Drink a glass of water.
* Apply mild pressure on the eyeballs.
* Swallow a teaspoon of honey or vinegar.
* Massage the roof of your mouth where it is soft and fleshy for about one minute.
* Swallow a small piece of crushed ice.
* Place an ice bag on the diaphragm just below the rib cage for several minutes.
* Drink a tablespoon of lemon juice.
* Lie on your left side for 10 to 15 minutes.
* Take a sniff of something with a strong aroma, such as vinegar.
* Chew activated charcoal tablets.

Did You Know...

Many breakfast cereals which advertise to be healthy are actually loaded with sugar?
Note the percentage of sucrose by weight of the following cereals:

All Bran: 20%
Bran Buds: 43.3%
Fortified Oat Flakes: 22.2%
Granola w/ almonds and filberts:21.4%
Heartland: 23.1%
Raisin Bran: 10.6%
Rice Krispies: 10%

What's WORSE!?
Apple Jacks: 55%
Cocoa Pebbles: 53.5%
Count Chocula: 44.2%
Crunch Berries: 43.4%
Froot Loops: 47.4%
Honeycomb: 48.4%
King Vitaman: 58.5%
Lucky Charms: 50.4%
Sugar Smacks: 61.3%
Trix: 46.6%

HIVES

Hives, or urticaria, is a skin condition characterized by a sudden outbreak of red, itchy raised skin blotches. Hives can occur anywhere on the body. Welts may vary in size from the diameter of a match head to rashes that cover large areas of the body.

The cause of hives is unknown in nine out of ten cases. Many cases are related to allergies triggering a histamine release. Many cases are also associated with stress or heavy metal toxicity. Severity of cases can vary greatly. If swelling occurs around the throat and interferes with breathing or swallowing, seek medical attention immediately.

The skin is a major part of the excretory system responsible for waste removal. If toxins are present in the body, the skin is one means of excretion. Hives and rashes may be the result.

What to do:

* Miserable as hives are, there is little one can do to relieve symptoms. If you know what the irritant is, remove it immediately.

* Cold water can help relieve itching.

* Calamine lotion may help relieve itching.

* Rub wheat germ oil over hives.

* Supplement raw adrenal glandulars which can assist in the production of anti-inflammatory hormones.

* Supplement nutrients and herbs which support the adrenal glands such as the B Complex, vitamin C chamomile, echinacea, ginseng, sarsparilla, licorice, etc.

* Avoid stress which can intensify breakouts.

* Colon cleansing, enemas or blood purifiers such as alfalfa are beneficial to help remove toxins from the body.

* You may wish to have an hair mineral analysis done to check for levels of toxicity.

Beneficial supplementation:

B Complex:
Vitamin C: 500-1,000 mg every hour until saturation level is reached.
Raw adrenal glandulars:
Herbs: Alfalfa, Caltrop, Chamomile, Echinacea, Ginseng, Licorice, Sarsparilla, and Yellow dock.

How to avoid:

Whenever possible, avoid items which you suspect as the cause of breakouts.
Avoid alcohol and processed foods which add stress on the body by depleting nutrients.
Alfalfa can be used as a preventative blood tonic. It cleanses the blood and helps keep the body free of toxins.

HYPERTENSION
(High Blood Pressure)

Hypertension is an abnormal elevation of blood pressure. Average blood pressure for men is 120/80, and slightly lower for females. Blood pressure which consistently exceeds 140/90 is considered high. The lower figure (diastolic) is usually considered the most important, because it is the pressure the arteries are under, even at rest.

Hypertension is a common disorder which often exists without symptoms and with unknown exact cause although in most cases diet is probably the most important factor.

The risk of hypertension is increased by overweight, high sodium chloride intake, high cholesterol level, stress, cigarette smoking, excessive use of stimulants, use of oral contraceptives and family history of high blood pressure.

Symptoms of hypertension may be nonexistent, or they may include headache, nervousness, insomnia, nosebleeds, blurred vision, edema, shortness of breath, dizziness, and ringing in the ears.

Presently, one-third of the American population suffers from hypertension. Because hypertension is one of the major contributors to cardiovascular disease, the number one cause of death in America, hypertension is now being examined more closely. There are a number of things which contribute to both these conditions from a dietary standpoint.

What to do:

* Most people can lower their blood pressure by eating less meat and more vegetables. The most effective way to lower blood pressure safely, rapidly, and permanently is an entirely vegetarian diet.

189

* A low fat and high fiber diet has shown to help control hypertension in a significant way. Polyunsaturated fats (Omega 3 fatty acids, fish oils, etc.) are also very important in helping to regulate blood pressure.

* Diet deficiencies have also been identified, and one survey conducted in 10 states over a two-year period showed that 70 percent of the study group was deficient in calcium, magnesium, iron, and vitamins A, C and B-6, all of which are beneficial to hypertension. These vitamins and minerals are cofactors which are needed by the enzyme systems of the body. They are of critical importance, in spite of the fact that they are not needed in large quantities.

* Individuals who are overweight and have hypertension can lower their blood pressure significantly by losing weight.

* Eliminate consumption of sodium chloride. Salt (sodium) has long been thought to be a major contributor to hypertension and, while more work is still needed, chloride, more so than sodium, is now believed to be a primary variable.

* Eliminate stress whenever possible. When an individual is under stress, one can suspect that vitamins B-1, B-2, B-6, B-12, C, and possibly magnesium, are all very, very low in the system. A number of these play a big part in the regulation of blood pressure. In general, stress tends to lower the resistance of the immune system allowing other things to enter the system.

* Hibiscus flowers seem to decrease the viscosity of the blood.

* Garlic, a time proven ancient remedy to reduce high blood pressure, among many things, may help to dissolve blood clots and reduce cholesterol, triglycerides, low-density lipoproteins, platelet aggregation and arterial plaque-all of which provide relief from chronic hypertension.

Suggested Supplementation:

B Complex:
Niacin:
Vitamin C: 3,000+ mg daily
Bioflavonoids:
Vitamin E: 100-600 IU daily
Calcium: 800 mg three times daily
Magnesium:
Potassium:
Silicon:
Flax Seed Oil:
Lecithin:
Fiber:
Herbs: Ceyenne (Capsicum), Garlic, Glucomannan, Hawthorn Berries, Hibiscus Flowers, Hops, Lady's Slipper, Passion Flower, Skullcap, and Valerian.

How to avoid:

Regular exercise is important in preventing high blood pressure because it keeps the circulatory system healthy.

Promoting a peaceful outlook on life is of primary importance to prevent hypertension.

HYPOGLYCEMIA

Hypoglycemia, or low blood sugar, is an abnormally low level of glucose in the blood. There are three types of hypoglycemia. Two of them are rare organic forms involving the pancreas: tumors of the pancreas and enlargement of the island of Langerhans. The most common form is functional hypoglycemia and is caused by an inadequate diet that is too high in refined carbohydrates that results in impaired absorption and assimilation of food ingested. An over consumption of carbohydrates causes the blood sugar level to rise rapidly, stimulating the pancreas to secrete an excess of insulin. This excess insulin removes too much sugar from the blood, resulting in an abnormally low blood sugar level.

An inadequate diet, such as one high in sugar or simple carbohydrates, stress, overwork, skipping meals, etc., can trigger the blood sugar level to drop, causing many of the following symptoms: Cravings for sugars or sweets, lack of stamina, fatigue, constant hunger, tendency to gain weight, allergies, caffeine cravings, muscle cramps or spasms, mood swings or irritability, nervous habits, insomnia, anxiety, blurred vision or dry eyes, depression or crying spells, frequent headaches, inability to concentrate or poor memory, light headed, dizzy, or faint feelings, feelings of inadequacy or loss of confidence, cold sweats, indigestion, uncomfortable menstrual periods, low sex drive, cold fingers or toes.

Symptoms are usually episodic, being related to the time and content of the previous meal. Symptoms are usually improved by eating.

Hypoglycemia is commonly associated with food allergies.

What to do:

* The therapeutic diet for hypoglycemia is high in protein, low in carbohydrates (unrefined complex) and moderate in fat. Carbohydrates should only include those which are slow absorbing such as vegetables, and whole-grain products. One should avoid all sugar and refined carbohydrates as well as products which contain them.
* Eat small frequent meals

Beneficial supplementation:

Vitamin A:
B Complex:
Niacin: 300-450 mg daily
Folic Acid:
Vitamin C: 1,000 mg three-five times daily
Vitamin E:
Magnesium:
Potassium:
Chromium: 200 mcg per day
Zinc:
Free-form or pre-digested amino acids:
Bee pollen:
Acidophilus:
Spirulina: one tsp three times daily
Lecithin:
Digestive enzymes:
Raw adrenal:
Raw pancreas:
Herbs: Alfalfa, Aloe Vera juice, Dandelion, Hawthorn, Juniper, Kelp, Licorice, Safflower, and Saffron.
Useful foods: Whole grains (especially oats and oat flour), nuts, raw milk products (if no sign of allergy exists), avocado, brewer's yeast, jerusalem artichokes.

How to avoid:

Avoid sugar (including fructose, sucrose, honey and all sweeteners), refined and simple carbohydrates in your diet.

Avoid alcohol, coffee, cigarettes, and other stimulants.

Avoid foods which are naturally high in sugar, such as dried fruits, figs, plums, and grapes. Eat bananas only in moderation.

Enjoy fruit only in moderation and preferably combined with protein. Avoid fruit and vegetable juices, or drink only two or three ounces at one time.

Avoid stress.

Did You Know...

All oranges are not orange?
Florida oranges are frequently green
when they are ripe and then dyed
orange to please customers.

IMMUNE DEFICIENCY

The immune system is essential for human survival. The immune system protects us from invaders such as yeasts, bacteria and viruses, but also fumes, chemicals, and substances such as alcohol, nicotine, caffeine, and obviously the common cold and flu, sore throat, cold sores, etc. Without a properly functioning immune system good health simply cannot be maintained.

We are all provided a genetically active immune system and an acquired immune response. This means part of our immunity is inherited and the rest is obtained through accumulated responses to foreign body exposures.

The principal organs of the immune system are the thymus, bone marrow, spleen, and lymphoid tissue (for example, the tonsils). The immune system also consists of the lymphatic vessels, lymph nodes, specialized white blood cells such as the B-cells, T-cells, (killer, helper, and suppressor), macrophage cells, and antibodies (also called immunoglobulins). Each has a different responsibility but they all function together.

Without optimal immune protection we are susceptible to conditions ranging from the common cold and flu, various stages of immune deficiency syndrome, cancer and even AIDS.

It is the responsibility of the immune system to protect us from these conditions. We may take immunity for granted until we are threatened with losing it. Research now shows that much of its efficacy may depend greatly upon ourselves.

General immune deficiency is experienced by all of us from time to time. This is largely due to stress, nutritional deficiencies, exposure to pathogens and general state of health by the individual.

Immune deficiency is characterized by:
Fatigue, loss of stamina and energy,
Swollen lymph nodes,
Frequent colds and infections,
Loss of appetite and weight loss,
Fever, night sweats,
Skin rashes and cold sores,
Diarrhea, etc.

These are due to the inability of the immune system to effectively fight off intruders such as the common cold, flu, bacteria, viruses, allergens, and even cancer.

The degree to which we are affected by immune deficiency depends on a number of factors, such as our general state of health and how we respond.

What to do:

* **Rest and relaxation:** Studies have shown that the immune system functions best while we are asleep. Deep sleep is important for immune function, for example, B-cell and macrophage activity increases. Some researchers even think of sleep as an aspect of immune function. The body needs to shut down in order for the immune system to effectively fight off what it has encountered. Most people know that we tend to sleep more when we are sick. It seems obvious that we must therefore need it. Lack of sleep, insomnia, and irregular sleeping habits (common with irregular work hours) have been shown to be detrimental to one's health and longevity.

* **Dietary changes:** Simple nutritious foods, soups, fresh fruits and vegetables and juices, and lots of liquids (particularly pure water), which help flush toxins, etc. out the body, are important to optimal health. Also, avoid processed foods, sugar, caffeine, alcohol and tobacco.

* **Attitude:** A positive attitude and desire for wellness is always of importance for optimal health.

* **Maintain proper hygiene.**

* **Avoid stress.**

* **Colostrum:** Both supplemental and from mother's milk contain immune support factors such as protein, immunoglobulins, antibodies, accessory factors, polypeptides, transforming growth factors, nucleotides, vitamins, etc. and are very beneficial to the immune system.

* **Nutritional Support:** Vitamin B Complex, vitamin C, E, and other nutritional support factors may be critical for speedy recovery. Dr. Linus Pauling, Ph.D., tells us the body requires large doses as high as 20-40+ grams of vitamin C per day in times of stress and illness.

* Vitamin C stimulates the production of interferon and increases the activity of certain WBC (white blood cells).

* Pantothenic acid (Vitamin B-5) is important to make antibodies and for normal adrenal functioning.

* Vitamin A alone can greatly increase the size and effectiveness of the thymus gland.

* Zinc, containing anti-bacterial/viral properties, is important for the health of the immune system.

* **Protein:** Consume an adequate amount of complete protein daily which is needed to make antibodies.

* **Anti-oxidants:** Vitamins C, A, and E, beta carotene, bioflavonoids, zinc, selenium, and CoQ10 are extremely important antioxidants which help prevent the formation of free radicals caused by pollutants in our air, food and water.

* **Herbal Suport:** Echinacea is a natural herbal antibiotic that counters the effects of most poisons in the body. It is the prime remedy to help the body rid itself of microbial infections. It is effective against both viral and bacterial attacks, not so by killing these organisms but by supporting the body's natural defense system.

Echinacea is a multi-faceted beneficial herb. It has a number of positive properties in the body. It is not geared to just one activity like many drugs are. Due to the chemical composition of echinacea, it has a number of different modes of action including: Antiseptic, antimicrobial, antisecretory, anti-inflammatory, antiphlogistic and vulnerary)

Echinacea acts similar to the manner in which

penicillin does. The chemical compounds responsible for this activity are called echinosides. In many cases, echinacea is more effective than the synthesized versions because it's activity is more broad-spectrum. In addition to the antibiotic property, it protects and supports the cells in other ways as well, for example, it has shown to be helpful to increase the production of white blood cells. Synthetic drugs are much more specific acting and therefore not as useful and supportive to the body.

Echinacea works extremely well in combination with other agents, such as vitamin C and garlic. Echinacea contains 17-18 percent vitamin C by dry weight in the form of bioflavonoids. If you add vitamin C to this, somehow the body assimilates the ascorbic acid more freely.

Suggested supplementation:

Vitamin A:
Beta Carotene:
B Complex:
Vitamin B-5:
Vitamin C:
Bioflavonoids:
Vitamin E:
Iron:
Selenium:
Zinc:
Essential Fatty Acids: Evening Primrose Oil, Flax
    Seed Oil, etc.
CoQ10:
Acidophilus:
Spirulina:
Colostrum:
    Maintenance: 1,000- 2,000 mg daily
    Therapeutic: 10,000 - 30,000 daily
Herbs: Alfalfa, Chaparral, Echinacea, Garlic, and Pau
    D'Arco.
In general: Blood purifiers, cleansing and tonics.

INDIGESTION

Indigestion (dyspepsia) is imperfect or incomplete digestion, manifesting itself in a sensation of fullness or discomfort in the abdomen accompanied by pains or cramps, heart burn, nausea, and gas. Headache, heart palpitations, and a disagreeable taste in mouth can also accompany indigestion.

Usually indigestion is the result of psychological stresses, anxiety, worry or disappointment disturbing the nervous mechanism that controls the contractions of stomach and intestinal muscles. Other causes are eating too rapidly (inadequate chewing), overeating, improper diet (overabundance in simple carbohydrates at the expense of other nutrients), unusual foods, fatty or spicy foods, swallowing large amount of air, or consuming stimulants (coffee, tea, or alcohol).

What to do:

* One's diet should be nutritionally well balanced and one should avoid eating when emotionally upset or overtired.

* Hydrochloric acid tablets may be helpful to breakdown foods as well as papaya enzymes.

* Peppermint has a soothing effect on the digestive tract and stimulates digestive secretion.

* Papaya (which contains papain) and pineapple (which contain bromelain) are beneficial digestive enzymes.

* Fennel is a natural remedy for gas and stomach acid. This herb can be sprinkled on food to prevent stomach gas.

* Anise seeds are beneficial for a sour stomach. The seeds can be chewed or ground and sprinkled on food.

* Mint tea (peppermint or spearmint) helps sooth the stomach.

* Activated charcoal can relieve stomach gas because it absorbs it like a sponge. It also can absorb intestinal bacteria which can cause gas. Charcoal is also good for diarrhea and hiccups.

Beneficial supplementation:

B Complex:
Hydrochloric acid:
Digestive enzymes:
 Betaine HCL
 Bromelain
 Papain
 Amylase
 Lipase
 Chymosin
 Trypsin
 Lisotozyme
Acidophilus:
Papaya
Pineapple juice:
Activated Charcoal:
Herbs: Anise, Fennel, Peppermint and Spearmint.

How to avoid:

Eat meals leisurely in a comfortable relaxing atmosphere. Don't gobble food and sit down while you eat.

Eat meals at regular intervals. This helps the stomach secrete digestive juices.

Do not water-log food.

Avoid large, heavy meals high in fat.

Drink papaya pineapple juice with each meal to promote digestion and combat excess stomach acid.

Take papaya tablets with each meal.

Avoid smoking before, during and after meals.

Avoid candy and gum which may stimulate stomach acid.

Make sure you rinse your dishes and silverware free of any soapy film which can cause digestive problems.

INSECT BITES

Allergic reactions to insect stings are life-threatening to many people. The allergic reactions include dizziness, nausea, diarrhea, itching and difficulty breathing. Offending insects are hornets, yellow jackets and wasps. The antidote is a vaccine made from insect venom which immunizes a person against the same type of insect.

What to do:

* Scrape out any stingers with your fingernail or a dull knife. Do not try to pull the stinger out. Squeezing will only inject more venom into the wound.
* Wash the bite wound with soap and water.
* Apply an ice pack and/or paste of baking soda and water to relieve the pain.
* Elevate area to reduce fluid retention and swelling.
* Take 1,000 mg vitamin C every hour until you reach saturation.

Beneficial supplementation:

Vitamin B-1:
Vitamin C: 1,000 mg every hour if stung by bee
Brewer's Yeast:
Herbs: Aloe Vera gel, Comfrey, Feverfew and Papaya for insect bites; Tea Tree Oil and Goldenseal as insect repellents.

How to avoid:

Be careful when outside cooking or eating. Food and drink often attract insect.

Don't wear open shoes or loose fitting clothes. Avoid bright colored clothing that may attract insects.

Wear bug proof clothing such as light weight, water proof rain gear of Gore-Tex, Klimate or coated nylon. These breathable fabrics are so tightly woven that bugs bounce off as easily as raindrops. The garments have tight closings at ankles, wrists and neck.

Do not wear perfume or hair spray lotions or any other cosmetics. They may attract insects.

Be careful when gardening. Wear a hat and long sleeved shirt, boots and gloves.

Tea Tree Oil and Goldenseal are natural insect repellents.

Feverfew is a good insect repellent. Mix three capsules of Feverfew into a 16 ounce spray bottle filled with cool distilled water. Shake well and spray over clothing and skin. This is also effective for pets.

Vitamin B-1 and Brewer's yeast also repel insects.

INSOMNIA

Insomnia is a difficulty in falling asleep, staying asleep, or inability to fall back to sleep.

The majority of cases of insomnia are caused by mental disturbances such as depression, an obsessive compulsive personality, anxiety, tension, physical pain, or discomfort. Overeating and indigestion are also common causes of insomnia. Insomnia may originate from the diet or faulty digestion resulting in vitamin, mineral, enzyme or amino acid deficiencies.

Deficiencies in the B vitamins (especially B-6 and B-12), vitamin C, protein, calcium, magnesium, and potassium have been associated with insomnia. Vitamins B-6 and C are needed for the conversion of tryptophan into serotonin in the brain. Magnesium is a common deficiency which can trigger over sensitivity to noise, light and other stimuli.

Medical problems such as hyper- or hypo-thyroid, asthma, allergies, heart disorders, poor circulation, ulcers, migraine headaches, arthritis, diabetes, kidney disease, epilepsy, etc., can also cause insomnia.

Heat, cold, humidity, noise, poor ventilation, an uncomfortable bed and other environmental factors can interfere with sleep.

Stimulants (sugar, caffeine, salt, ephedra, etc.) interfere with sleep as well as some depressants (alcohol, antihistamines, etc.).

What to do:

* If a nutrient deficiency is responsible for the problem, one needs to correct the deficiency.
* Warm showers and baths are relaxing for the body and nerves.
* A hot footbath with chamomile or other relaxing tea will help produce sleep.

* Do relaxation exercises or meditation before going to bed.

* The amino acid tryptophan is necessary to sleep because it converts to serotonin (the sleep chemical) in the brain. Foods high in tryptophan include turkey, milk, cheese, and other dairy products. You may try eating these foods an hour before bedtime. One of the classic remedies for insomnia is to drink a glass of warm milk before bedtime.

* Inositol also converts to tryptophan once it gets inside the blood brain barrier.

* If insomnia is stress related, exercise during the day to relieve tension.

Beneficial supplementation:

B Complex:
Vitamin B-6: 10-100 mg
Vitamin B-12: 25 mg
Inositol: 1-10 grams before bedtime
Niacin: 100 mg-2 grams
Pantothenic Acid: 100 mg
Vitamin C: 1-5 grams daily
Vitamin D: 2,000 IU
Vitamin E: 400 IU
Calcium: 2 grams
Magnesium: 500 mg
Phosphorus:
Potassium:
Herbs: Catnip, Chamomile, Hops, Lady's Slipper, Skullcap, and Valerian Root.

How to avoid:

Try to go to bed at approximately the same time every night and get up at the same time every morning. If you do not fall asleep in 20 minutes, get out of bed and do something relaxing.

Avoid coffee or other stimulants.

Reduce salt intake.

Avoid drinking alcohol before bedtime.

Keep the bedroom cool: 64-66 degrees.

Do not work or watch T.V. in the bedroom. Use the bedroom primarily for sleeping.

Get exercise and fresh air regularly.

Did You Know...

Too much coffee can contribute to osteoporosis later in life? Coffee can cause a loss of calcium and magnesium which presents a threat to women especially.

ITCHING

Itching, a feeling that makes one want to scratch, is caused by irritation and starvation of the nerve endings which causes inflammation. Itching can occur anywhere, the scalp, nose, eyes, feet and toes, hands and fingers, rectum, genitalia, etc. A number of conditions are associated with itching: itchy scalp (seborrheic dermatitis or dandruff, etc.), psoriasis, eczema, hives, rashes, hemorrhoid itching, or any other condition, commonly known as pruritus.

Irritation can be caused by numerous things including allergens, chemical irritants, nutritional or chemical imbalances, pre-existing conditions, strain on the adrenal glands, etc.

Strain on the adrenal glands causes them to use nutrients very rapidly so the adrenals are no longer capable of producing a balance of hormones and chemicals. They instead tend to produce nervous adrenalin which causes a constriction or narrowing of the blood vessels and capillaries leading to the extremities such as the scalp, hands, feet, etc.

Itching may be a signal that your adrenal glands are overburdened and are not receiving the nutrients it needs.

Treatment is geared to the cause if it is known.

What to do:

* For topical chemical or allergic irritation, wash the area immediately with cool water. Try not to scratch, which can cause secondary infection and spread the infected area.
* As a natural antihistamine, take 1,000 mg vitamin C hourly until you reach saturation level.
* Take 60 milligrams of iron three times a day.
* Add apple cider vinegar to your bath.
* Try a cool shower or cold packs.
* Calamine lotion may relieve some types of itching to

a degree.
* Apply vitamin E cream directly to area
* Increase your intake of essential fatty acids, for example, flax seed oil, evening primrose oil, etc.
* For dry skin itching, take a lukewarm bath with bath oil.

Beneficial supplementation:

B Complex:
Vitamin B-5 (Pantothenic acid): 100 mg one to three times daily.
Vitamin C: 1,000 mg hourly
Acidophilus:
Essential Fatty Acids: (Flax seed, Evening Primrose oil, etc.
Herbs: Yarrow

How to avoid:

Avoid known allergens and irritants.
Avoid sugar and other refined simple carbohydrates.

KIDNEY STONES

Kidney stones (renal calculi) are abnormal accumulations of mineral salts, which form in the kidney but lodge anywhere in the urinary tract. They can be as small as sand or gravel or as large as bird eggs which would be large enough to block the ureter tube and stop the flow of urine. The stones are composed primarily of calcium phosphate or oxalate. If surgically removed, they may reappear if the diet has not improved.

Kidney stones may be present without symptoms, or one may experience intermittent, dull, dragging pain in the low back, testicle, groin, or leg which is usually aggravated by movement. Hemorrhage (bleeding) and renal colic (a sharp pain in the lower back and groin) occur when a stone enters the ureter, which can last or hour or days. Pallor, frequency of urination, nausea, vomiting and agony may occur.

Causes include deficiencies in magnesium, calcium, vitamins A, B-6, or D, excesses in phosphorus, dairy products, oxalic acid (chocolate, cocoa, tea, spinach, rhubarb, chard, and beet tops), alkaline, purines (as in gout), sugar, or coffee. Stress, a diet low in protein (which draw out calcium from the bone), excess fluid loss, chronic urinary infections, and hypercalcuria (too much calcium in the urine) also can contribute to kidney stone formation.

What to do:

As with other conditions one needs to determine the cause before the best treatment can be determined. For example, one should not take high doses of vitamin B-6 if one does not have a deficiency. With prolonged high doses, vitamin B-6 can be toxic.

* Magnesium helps keep calcium in solution and mobilizes calcium from the stone. Small daily doses of magnesium oxide seem to forestall the formation of

211

calcium-oxalate lumps, which are by far the most prevalent kind of kidney stone.

   * Limit protein intake to 70 grams per day.

   * Avoid refined foods which are commonly low in potassium and high in salt. These foods, combined with a diet low in fruits and vegetables, make the urine too alkaline which prevents minerals from being held in solution and cause them to deposit as stones.

Beneficial supplementation:

Vitamin A:
B Complex:
Vitamin B-6: 50-200 mg twice daily, (if deficient, total of 1,000 mg daily)
Vitamin E:
Magnesium: 100 mg two to four times a day.

How to avoid:

Maintain proper dietary calcium-phosphorous ratio.

Diet should include plenty of fresh vegetables, fruit, legumes, whole grains, and fermented dairy products.

Avoid excess aspirin.

LEG CRAMPS
(Charley Horse)

Leg cramps (involuntary painful contraction or spasm of a muscle in the leg or foot) are an extremely common and disturbing problem. Cramps commonly occur at night, when the limbs are cool, particularly after a day of exertion. Cramps occur more frequently in the elderly, the young, and persons with arteriosclerosis. The cramps may be triggered by an unnatural position which impairs the blood supply to the lower extremities. Cramps which occur while walking are more serious than those which occur while resting.

Leg cramps may be signaling nutritional deficiencies, most commonly calcium, which is necessary for normal muscle contraction. Other deficiencies include thiamine, pantothenic acid, biotin, vitamin C, and magnesium.

Sodium loss, such as with heavy perspiration or diarrhea, may result in muscle cramps.

A charley horse usually occurs in the quadriceps or hamstring muscle in the back of the thigh. It is the result of a pulled and bruised muscle which results in stiffness and soreness. It is usually caused by a blow or a forceful stretch of the leg during athletic activity. Additional protein may be required to help rebuild damaged tissue.

What to do:

* The discomfort of a leg cramp can often be relieved by walking or moving the leg.

Beneficial supplementation:

B Complex:
B-1 (Thiamine):
Pantothenic acid: 100 mg
Biotin:

213

Vitamin C: Up to saturation level
Bioflavonoids: 300-1,000 mg daily
Vitamin E: 400-1,000 IU one to three times daily
Calcium: 1,000-1,500 mg daily
Magnesium: 500-1,000 mg daily
Phosphorus:
Sodium:
Protein:
Essential Fatty Acids:

How to avoid:

Maintain adequate intake of calcium and magnesium.
Maintain adequate levels of moderate exercise.

MEMORY

Memory is the ability or power that enables one to remember and recall, through unconscious means of association, previous sensations, impressions, ideas, concepts, and all information that has been consciously learned.

Poor memory can be a natural part of aging (free radical damage, for example) or can be symptoms of an underlying cause such as nutrient deficiencies (B Complex and amino acids especially) alcoholism, hypoglycemia (low blood sugar) or Alzheimer's Disease.

Alzheimer's Disease is a form of brain disease which leads to confusion, memory loss, restlessness, trouble moving, speech difficulties, etc. The disease often starts in late mid-life with slight defects in memory and behavior. The exact cause is unknown, but high levels of aluminum have been found in brain tissue of affected individuals. Good nutrition may slow progress of the disease.

What to do:

* Choline, a member of the B Complex family is one of the few substances that penetrate the blood brain barrier, which normally protects the brain against variations in the daily diet, and goes directly into the brain cells to produce a chemical that aids memory. It also aids in the sending of nerve impulses, specifically those in the brain used in the formation of memory.

* Eat more foods which contain choline:
Egg yolks
Brain
Heart
Green leafy vegetables
Yeast
Liver
Wheat germ
Lecithin.

215

* Manganese, important for normal central nervous system function, can help improve memory, and also help eliminate fatigue and reduce nervous irritability. Manganese helps stabilize acetylcholine so it is not prematurely used or discharged.

* Ginkgo Biloba Leaf extract is one of the latest breakthrough discoveries in the science of brain nutrition. It has been shown to be a powerful free radical scavenger and inhibitor. It also has been shown in several clinical trials to significantly decrease the symptoms of impaired brain blood flow, including poor short term memory and decreased attention span.

* Glutamine, which passes through the blood brain barrier, is used as a fuel for the brain and which also helps keep excess amounts of ammonia from damaging the brain and helps to focus our thinking.

* Tyrosine stimulates the production of norepinephrine, the "alertness" brain chemical, and has a role in sharpening learning, memory and awareness, and elevated mood and motivation.

* Taurine and methionine help nourish brain cells and help choline's effect in promoting thinking ability. It also helps stabilize brain cell membranes, minimizing agitation, restlessness, inability to focus, (an extreme form of this is epilepsy).

* Zinc is a co-enzyme with vitamin B-6 , which is needed to make all the major neurotransmitters, except acetylcholine.

* Magnesium is extremely important for the brain; it supports the brain in producing energy as ATP. Once the body makes ATP, it immediately combines with magnesium to stabilize and store it. The B vitamins require manganese or magnesium as their co-enzymes to work properly.

* Supplementation with tonic herbs such as Ginseng, Astragalus, or Dong Quai, either alone or in combination are beneficial for individuals who are in a malnourished weakened state. It is also helpful for preventing symptoms of aging including poor memory. For superior results, tonic herbs are combined with foods at mealtime.

* American Ginseng combined with Red Deer Antler

(equal parts) is known as the most powerful energy-memory tonic for individuals of all ages.

* Siberian Ginseng also has endurance-giving properties, and is known as an adaptogen, assists in the endurance of high levels of stress. (Using the brain all the time is a form of stress.)

* The herb Calamus is highly regarded in Ayurvedic medicine as an herb that promotes wisdom by improving mental focus.

* Gotu Cola is a classic memory herb for brain fatigue.

* Ginger and cayenne are good for stimulation of circulation.

Beneficial supplementation:

B Complex: 50 mg twice daily
Vitamin B-1:
Choline: 3,000 mg daily in divided doses
Magnesium:
Manganese:
Zinc:
L-glutamine: 500 mg three times daily
Methionine:
Taurine:
Tyrosine:
Lecithin:
DMAE-H3: 10-25 drops daily
Herbs: Astragalus, Calamus, Cayenne, Dong Quai,
    Ginkgo Biloba Leaf Extract, Ginger, Ginseng
    (American and Siberian), Gota Kola, and Red Deer
    Antler.

Did You Know...

Frozen orange juice concentrate may lose its vitamin C? Frozen orange juice mixed with water from copper pipes may lose its vitamin C. Heavy mineralized water (such as water sitting in copper pipes) destroys vitamin C. Mix frozen juices with pure bottled water or run the tap for two or three minutes before using the water.

MENTAL HEALTH

The importance of a sound, well-functioning brain for health and happiness cannot be overstated. The brain is the master control bio-computer of the human organism. It generates every thought and mood. It controls our movements, regulates our breathing, heartbeat, body temperature, and hormone balance.

Yet in spite of the absolute importance of a smooth running brain for health and vitality, the brain is usually the most poorly nourished organ in the human body.

The brain weighs about three pounds-less than two percent of our total body weight-yet uses 20 percent of the body's total energy supply. The estimated 10 billion-plus neurons (brain cells) have a voracious appetite for fuel (sugar), oxygen, vitamins, minerals, amino acids, and fatty acids, which **must** be satisfied every minute of every day of our lives. All these nutrients must be delivered to the brain constantly by our bloodstream. If the blood flow to the brain is interrupted even for 15-20 seconds, unconsciousness results. If deprived of blood or oxygen for more than five-ten minutes, the brain dies.

Only slight changes in the molecular amounts of numerous chemicals can bring on changes in the brain affecting behavior, mood, and perception. Medical professionals have found that using megavitamin therapy for many mental disorders has doubled recovery rates.

Mental illness as a physical disease can result from low brain concentrations of vitamin B-1, B-6, B-12, niacin, pantothenic acid, folic acid, vitamin C, various minerals (especially zinc) and amino acids.

Psychological problems can also stem from undetected allergies, (such as milk, wheat or corn) or from excess copper, aluminum or other metals in the body.

About 30 percent of schzophrenics are deficient in vitamin B-6 and zinc. This condition is referred to as pyroluria and has had good results with.Vitamin B-6, zinc and magnesium supplementation. Major symptoms of pyroluria include withdrawal and depression. Other

219

indications are as follows:

Breath or body odor.
Intolerance to some proteins, alcohol or drugs.
Morning nausea and constipation.
Crowded upper front teeth.
White spots on fingernails.
Difficulty in remembering dreams.
Pale skin that does not tolerate sunlight.
Frequent abdominal pain.
Frequent head colds and infections.
Stretch marks.
Irregular menstrual cycle or impotency.

What to do:

* Avoid sugar. Research shows that 75 percent of patients suffering from anxiety and panic disorders had a dramatic increase in anxiety after eating as little as one candy bar daily. Sugar causes the body to release adrenalin, which is the major factor in panic attacks, and also causes a draining of many of the nutrients required by the brain for optimal functioning.

* Avoid caffeine which releases adrenalin in the body.

* Avoid all recreational drugs, including alcohol.

* Practice deep breathing from the diaphragm. This causes the parasympathetic nervous system to take charge over the sympathetic nervous system.

Beneficial supplementation:

Vitamin B-1:
Vitamin B-6: 50-500 mg twice daily
Vitamin B-12:
Niacin:
Pantothenic acid:
Folic acid:
Vitamin C:
Manganese: 10 mg twice daily
Zinc gluconate:30 mg twice daily
Herbs: Cayenne, Ginseng, Gotu Kola

MORNING SICKNESS

Morning sickness is the term used to describe the feeling of nausea that occurs (often in the morning, but can occur throughout the day) in the early weeks of pregnancy. The exact cause is unknown besides the general physical changes due to the pregnancy. It may be necessary to clean the body to eliminate toxins that can cause nausea in pregnancy.

What to do:

* Relief is often received by eating frequent, small easily digested meals and not allowing the stomach to be empty. **NOTE:** Skipping meals (especially breakfast) can harm the fetus. Going without a meal can lower blood sugar levels and raise levels of fatty acids. These acids and other metabolic products can pass through the placenta and harm the fetus.
* Eat something (such as tea and crackers) in the morning before getting out of bed.
* Many women have reported that daily supplementation of vitamin B-6 has given them relief.
* Ginger Root capsules which are commonly used for motion sickness are also beneficial for morning sickness.
* The amino acid methionine has been effectively used to aid toxemia in pregnancy to prevent nausea.
* Red Raspberry or Peppermint tea often overcome nausea. Also beneficial may be Alfalfa, Catnip tea or Ginger tea.
* An ancient remedy for morning sickness is to grind lentils into a powder and take two teaspoons with rice cereal three times daily.

Beneficial supplementation:

Vitamin B-6: Do not exceed 75-100 mg daily
Methionine:
Herbs: Alfalfa, Catnip (tea), False Unicorn Root,
Fennel, Ginger Root (capsules or tea), Goldenseal,
Kelp, Peppermint (tea), and Red Raspberry (tea).

MOTION SICKNESS

Motion sickness is a condition caused by uneven or rhythmic motions in any combination of directions. Severe cases are characterized by nausea, vomiting, dizziness, and headache. Mild cases are characterized by headache and general discomfort.

Prevention of motion sickness is easier than the cure after symptoms are present.

What to do:

* Move to an area where there is less motion. In a car, this would be the front seat looking straight ahead. In an airplane, select a seat over a wing. On a ship, stay in the middle section on a deck rather than below.

* Look ahead at the horizon or close your eyes if watching passing scenery makes you ill.

* Lie in a semi-reclined position and keep your head as still as possible.

* Focus on something other than motion. For example, occupy yourself with reading or drawing instead of looking out the window.

Beneficial supplementation:

B Complex: 100 mg
Vitamin B-1:
Vitamin B-6: 75 mg daily
Herbs: Alfalfa, Catnip (tea), False Unicorn Root, Fennel, Ginger Root (capsules or tea), Goldenseal, Kelp, Peppermint (tea), and Red Raspberry (tea).

How to avoid:

Take two Ginger Root capsules thirty minutes to an hour before traveling. It generally does not provide relief after the onset of symptoms.

Vitamins B-1 and B-6 are effective when taken starting the day before you leave for the trip.

B Complex is also effective taken the day and the morning before you leave.

MOSQUITO BITES

A mosquito bite is a bite of a small flying bloodsucking insect. It may result in a severe allergic reaction in an allergic person, infection or, most often, an itching sore. Mosquitoes are carriers of many infectious diseases including encephalitis (inflammation of the brain) and yellow fever.

Mosquitoes are attracted by moisture, carbon dioxide, estrogens, sweat, or warmth.

How to avoid:

* Supplement and eat foods high in vitamin B-1, such as brown rice, brewer's yeast, wheat germ, blackstrap molasses and fish. Studies show that individuals who took vitamin B-1 supplements had fewer mosquito bites than individuals who did not. Vitamin B-1 can be depleted by an excess intake of sugar and alcohol.

* Eliminate refined sugar from your diet and in time (up to one year) mosquitoes will leave you alone. Sugar causes the skin to let off a sweet smell that attracts mosquitoes. When sugar is eliminated, the skin no longer produces this scent.

* Apply a few drops of Tea Tree Oil, a natural insecticide, which keeps mosquitoes as well as other bugs away.

* Spray Feverfew and water mixture over clothing and skin as a natural insect repellent.

Beneficial supplementation:

Vitamin B-1:
Tea Tree Oil:

Did You Know...

Many foods contain hidden sulfites? Most people now realize that salad bars and dried fruit contain added sulfites, but numerous other products also contain sulfites:

Baked goods: Cookies, crackers (even grahams), pie and quiche crusts, waffles, and wheat tortillas.

Beverages: Beer, cider, colas, fruit drinks and juices, instant tea, soup, vegetables juices, wine coolers and wine.

Candy, deserts, and syrups: Sugar, brown sugar, jams, jellies, pancake syrups, shredded coconut, gelatin, and fruit pie fillings.

Fish: Clams, crab, dried cod, lobster, scallops, shrimp, and canned seafood soups.

Fruits and vegetables: mushrooms, grapes, prepared salads, shredded cabbage, dried fruits, trail mixes, breakfast cereals containing dried fruits, dried fruit snacks or dietetic processes fruits.

Pasta, grains, and other carbohydrates: Spinach pasta, cornstarch, modified food starch, breadings, noodle and rice mixes, potato chips, and processed potato salad.

Relishes, condiments, and mixes: Horseradish, pickles, olives, onion relish, wine vinegar, pickled vegetables, sauerkraut, coleslaw, guacamole, gravies, and dried soup mixes.

NOTE: Added sulfites are not always listed on ingredient labels.

NAIL PROBLEMS

Nails are composed almost entirely of protein. Abnormal or unhealthy nails may be the result of a local injury, a glandular deficiency such as hypothyroidism or a deficiency of certain nutrients.

A protein deficiency can cause opaque white bands to appear on the nails or cause them to become dry, thin and brittle. Insufficient amounts of complete proteins and/or vitamin A slow down the rate of nail growth.

A shortage of vitamin A, iron, or calcium in the diet may also cause dryness and brittleness.

A lack of the B vitamins causes nails to become fragile, with horizontal or vertical ridges appearing.

A vitamin C, folic acid, protein deficiency may be indicated by frequent hangnails. An iron deficiency can disturb the growth of nails causing dryness, brittleness, thinning, flattening, and eventually the appearance of moon-shaped nails.

A zinc deficiency is often indicated by white spots on the nails.

What to do:

* **For brittle nails:** Keep them well moisturized. Avoid nail polish and nail polish remover. Buffing nails smooths them and keeps them free of debris. Avoid contact with detergent and chemicals. Iron supplementation may help. Foods high in iron include dark, green leafy vegetables, fish, legumes, and whole grains.

* **For hangnails:** Do not pull or tear; cut off with a sharp scissors. Proper moisturizing and wearing gloves whole doing work is the best way to prevent. Make sure diet includes sufficient amounts of vitamin C, folic acid and protein. **NOTE:** Gelatin is a poor source of protein for the nails.

* Vitamin A helps to prevent splitting nails.

227

* Supplement the diet with nutrients that may be beneficial.

* Raw potato juice and Horsetail herb are high in silica.

Beneficial supplementation:

Vitamin A: 25,000 IU once daily six days a week after any meal.

B Complex: 100 mg once daily

Folic Acid:

Vitamin C:

Calcium:

Iron:

Silica:

Zinc: 25-50 mg daily

Protein:

Herbs: Horsetail

NASAL CONGESTION
(Sinusitis)

Nasal congestion occurs when blood vessels in the nose enlarge, taking up space in the nasal cavity. This restricts the amount of air allowed in for easy breathing.

A common cold can lead to sinusitis, which is an acute inflammation of the accessory nasal sinuses with nasal congestion and postnasal discharge. Sinusitis is often accompanied by headache, pain behind the eye, tenderness, fever, and loss of smell.

Nasal congestion and sinusitis may be due to an inadequate diet (excess milk and dairy products, milk allergy, excess carbohydrates, raw vegetable deficiency, etc.) food or inhalant allergies, cold or flu virus, stress, or adrenal exhaustion.

Sinuses are air-containing spaces located within the skull. There function is tied in to the immune system. The membranes within them secrete mucus, and, within these secretions are ingredients that clean out the sinuses and nasal passages protecting us from infection.

When the nasal passages are irritated (by smoke, pollution, allergies, etc), the membranes secrete a lot more mucus to clean out the sinuses. Usually sinusitis develops when the individual has a cold or upper respiratory infection. This sets up an inflammatory condition of the nose and sinus cavities that obstructs the flow of secretions causing infection and more secretions. It something is not done to break the cycle, it gets worse and worse.

What to do:

* Eating hot soup speeds the flow of mucus out of the nose. Adding cayenne pepper and raw onion may hasten relief.

* Place eucalyptus leaves in a pot of boiling water for

229

five minutes. Turn the heat off and, with a towel draped over your head, lean over the pot and breathe in the herbal vapors. Be careful not to burn yourself.

* Try taking 500-1,000 mg of vitamin C every hour until you reach saturation. Vitamin C acts as a natural antihistamine, anti-inflammatory agent and helps fight infection.

* Vitamin C and protein help restore damaged sinus membrane tissue.

* Adequate intake of vitamin A, which helps maintain the health of the mucus membranes of the nose and throat, can help in the treatment of sinusitis.

* Vitamin A, potassium, calcium, and zinc (which is necessary for vitamin A mobilization from the liver, aid the work of the cilia in the nasal passageways that help the expulsion of mucus.

* Avoid the use of nasal decongestants (sprays, drops and inhalers). They work by shrinking swollen blood vessels in the nose. In time, vessels tend to "tire," making congestion worse.

* Chewing honeycomb is an ancient remedy for sinusitis.

* Glandulars such as raw thymus can help stimulate the immune system and raw adrenal can help stimulate production of anti-inflammatory hormones.

Beneficial supplementation:

Vitamin A: 25,000 IU up to six times a day in acute
    cases
B complex: 25-50 mg two to three times daily
Vitamin B-6: 100 mg twice daily
Vitamin C: 500-1,000 mg hourly in acute cases
Vitamin E:
Potassium:
Calcium:
Zinc:
Protein:
Garlic: two capsules three times daily
Onion: cooked and raw

230

Onion syrup: One tsp per hour in acute cases
Raw Adrenal:
Raw Thymus: One to four tablets per hour in acute
cases
Herbs: Comfrey, Coneflower (Echinacea
angustifolium), Eucalyptus, Fenugreek, and
Magnolia Blossoms (tea).

How to avoid:

Avoid abrupt changes in temperature.

Stay clear of household aerosol sprays.

Keep your oven clean (smoke can trigger congestion).

Have regular dental checkups (tooth infections spread easily into the sinuses).

Avoid known allergens.

Avoid dry heat-use a humidifier or vaporizer, especially in the bedroom, if it is hot and dry.

Avoid cigarettes and alcohol which are both irritating to the nasal passageways.

Eat a balanced diet and get plenty of exercise.

NERVOUSNESS

Nervousness, a feeling of tension, unease, anxiousness and excitability, can be caused by a large variety of circumstances and conditions. Overwork, lack of sleep, stress, poor diet, lack of exercise and fresh air may be only a few causes of nervousness.

What to do:

* To relieve nervous tension, massage the web structure of the hand between the finger and thumb. Apply hand cream for lubrication, and start massaging the left hand first. After five minutes switch to the right hand. The webbing between the thumb and fingers contain many nerve endings which when massaged is very relaxing to the entire body.
* Deep breathing exercises are also very beneficial to relieve nervous tension:
  1. While standing, place both hands high on the rib cage as near the arm pits as possible.
  2. Press inward as far as possible with both hands at the same time, exhaling through the open mouth.
  3. Suddenly release both hands at the same time.
  4. Inhale deeply holding the breath for five seconds. Repeat this exercise three to six times.
* Hot and cold fomentations, to the spine, stomach, liver and spleen are very beneficial for nervous people.

Beneficial supplementation:

B Complex:
Vitamin B-6:
Vitamin B-12:
Niacin:
PABA:
Vitamin C:

Calcium:

Magnesium:

Herbs: Betony, Catnip, Chamomile, European Vervain, Hops, Lady's Slipper, Mistletoe, Passion Flower, Pulsatilla, Red Sage (for nervous headache), Skullcap, and Valerian.

NIGHT BLINDNESS

Night blindness (nyctalopia) is a condition where a person can see well in daylight but not in fading or dim light. Night blindness is often due to a deficiency of vitamin A. Vitamin A deficiency can also cause additional eye problems including: Inability to adjust to darkness, blood-shot eyes, inflammation, burning sensations and sties.

What to do:

* Night blindness (as well as other eye problems) can often be aided or prevented by supplementing the diet with 2,500 to 7,500 IU of vitamin A a day.
* Heavy alcohol use appears to interfere with the liver's ability to store and release vitamin A into the system. Heavy drinkers should supplement their diet with vitamin A.

Beneficial supplementation:

Vitamin A: 2,500 to 7,500 IU daily.
Beta Carotene: (Safer form of vitamin A when higher doses are desired.)
Vitamin B-2:
Herbs: Bilberry

How to avoid:

Maintain adequate levels of vitamin A. Vitamin A is found in fish, liver, egg yolks, butter, cream, green leafy or yellow vegetables.
Avoid heavy alcohol use.

Did You Know...

Oral Contraceptives can interfere with the availability of vitamins? Vitamins C, B-1, B-6, B-12, and folic acid are common deficiencies amongst women on the pill.

OSTEOPOROSIS

Osteoporosis is a loss of normal bone density, marked by thinning of bone tissue and the growth of small holes in the bone. It occurs most frequently in women who have gone through menopause, individuals who are inactive or paralyzed and in individuals taking steroid hormones.

Osteoporosis may be painful (especially in the lower back), may cause frequent broken bones, loss of body height, and deformities (for example, hump-back look in elderly).

Estrogen (female sex hormone) is often used to prevent postmenopausal osteoporosis, but use of the hormone has risk of causing uterine cancer.

A major cause of osteoporosis is an inadequate intake of calcium over a period of years. The Minimum Daily Requirement for calcium for adults is 800 mg per day, while many people, especially the aged, get only 450 mg per day. It is estimated that over 30 percent of the American population suffers from calcium deficiency. In addition, calcium needs increase with age. Women who have passed menopause may need as much as 1,500 mg daily.

Other causes of osteoporosis are inability to absorb sufficient calcium through the intestines, calcium-phosphorus imbalance, lack of exercise, or lack of certain hormones.

What to do:

A diet that is adequate in protein, calcium, magnesium, phosphorus, vitamin C, and vitamin D is the best treatment and prevention for osteoporosis.

A calcium supplement is necessary to rebuild lost bone tissue and prevent further loss. Calcium lactate, calcium gluconate, calcium hydroxyapatite, or chelated calcium are the best supplemental sources.

Eat foods which are high in calcium: Milk and milk products, fish, eggs, cereal products, beans, many types of nuts and seeds, fruit (especially oranges and papaya), and vegetables (especially green leafy). (Meat contains calcium but is not a good source to rely upon because it can actually contribute to a calcium deficiency.)

* One cup lowfat yogurt contains 350-450 milligrams calcium.
* One cup skim milk contains 300-350 milligrams calcium.
* One ounce colby cheese contains about 293 milligrams calcium.
* 10 dried figs contain about 270 milligrams calcium.
* One cup rhubarb contains about 120 milligrams calcium.
* One-half cup almonds contains about 160 milligrams calcium.
* One-third pound salmon contains about 120 milligrams calcium.
* One cup broccoli contains about 140 milligrams calcium.
* Three and one-half ounces tofu has about 100 milligrams calcium.
* One tablespoon of blackstrap molasses has about 140 milligrams calcium.

Calcium Facts:

* 80 percent of all American women are calcium deficient.
* Men and women over age 30 require up to 67 percent more calcium than do 16 year olds.
* According to "The Calcium Bible" by Patricia Hausman, M.S., calcium is not only essential as a bone-building nutrient, but also shows promise as one which helps control blood pressure.
* Calcium is important to assist in vitamin absorption as well as help with nerve, hormone and enzyme functioning.
* Due to stress, bad eating habits and lack of exercise, the mineral we are most likely to be low

in is calcium.
* Calcium deficiency can lead to nervousness, fatigue, muscle cramping, menstrual problems, periodontal disease, high blood pressure, and particularly osteoporosis.
* Research findings reveal that the time of day you take a calcium supplement is vital for maximizing its absorption, and the most effective time is nighttime.
* The form of the calcium taken and which co-nutrients it is taken with are important in achieving the most beneficial results from a calcium supplement. Vitamin D (particularly D-3) is needed for optimal calcium absorption. Foods rich in vitamin D include milk, salmon, tuna, and sardines.

Some experts believe that a calcium deficiency is actually caused by a magnesium deficiency which requires magnesium supplementation.

Other experts say the answer to bone problems is silica. People who do not get enough calcium, but have no bone problems, may be consuming large amounts of silica. When a baby is born, the ratio of calcium to silica is very different from the ratio of an older person. This may be why babies' bones are so resilient. Silica is actually a youth factor. With the loss of silica, bones become older, and more brittle.

This is in accord with one of the conclusions of the osteoporosis symposium, which demonstrated that changes in the elasticity of bone result in a greater propensity to fracture. Bone growth involves the process of adding calcium for hardness, plus increasing collagen, the tough connective tissue that binds everything together and gives bones flexibility. Silica is essential for both these processes.

An important study conducted at the School of Public Health at the University of California, Los Angeles, (UCLA), shows that silica-supplemented bones have a 100 percent increase in collagen over low-silica bones. "If you do not have enough calcium and silica, your body leaches the calcium from your bones for tissue needs."

Silica is important in the following ways:
* In the formation and repair of bone, cartilage, skin and connective tissues of all kinds.
* As a participant in several metabolic processes.
* As an essential nutrient in the initial calcification of bones in newborns.
* As a corrective dietary supplement in skeletal abnormalities resulting from silica deficiency.
* In producing effects totally independent of the presence of vitamin D, but synergistic with ascorbate.

Silica is present in the body as free soluble monosilic acid. Connective tissues such as the aorta, trachea, tendon, bone and skin are usually rich in silica. Silica is found as an integral part of the collagen and their protein complexes. It is crucial to the formation of bones and cartilage matrices, both intracellularly. Apparently, silica works by not stimulating cell proliferation, but by actual participation in cell formation. Thus silica plays an important metabolic role in connective tissue formation, and also becomes a crucial structural component of such tissue. During the aging process, connective tissue changes rapidly. Not surprisingly, silica concentration in these tissues steadily declines. Nothing is known yet about possible cause and effect relationships, but it is possible that cellular silica levels and aging are closely related.

Another expert tells us that in the body silica converts into calcium.

As mentioned earlier, proper stomach acidity is required for calcium to dissolve. If you are not sure you have adequate stomach acidity, try taking this old folk remedy with your calcium supplement: One tablespoon vinegar mixed with one tablespoon honey.

Another suggestion is to take a hydrochloric acid supplement with calcium if you are not sure you have adequate stomach acidity.

Beneficial supplementation:

Vitamin B-12: 30-900 mcg daily
Vitamin C: 1,000-2,000 mg two to four times daily
Vitamin D: 5,000 IU daily
Vitamin E: 600 IU daily
Calcium: 1-2 grams daily
Magnesium: 500-1,000 mg daily
Copper:
Fluoride:
Phosphorus:
Silica:
Protein:
Herbs: Comfrey and Horsetail.

How to avoid:

Make sure you are getting a sufficient supply of calcium in your diet.

Avoid eating a diet high in animal protein which induces a calcium deficiency.

Avoid eating sweets and refined carbohydrates which stimulate alkaline digestive juices, making calcium insoluble.

Avoid prolonged stress, alcohol abuse, antibiotics, steroids, and cigarettes. Tobacco leaches calcium from the bones.

Make sure you get adequate exercise.

PAIN

Pain is an unpleasant sense caused by signals from some sense nerve endings. Pain is a basic symptom of inflammation and is an important clue to the cause of many disorders.

Chronic pain is often associated with depression, which in turn can make the pain worse.

What to do:

* Cold is the best remedy for the pain of injury. Applying ice will provide the following benefits:
* Ice numbs the affected area of pain.
* Ice decreases swelling by cutting down the blood supply.
* Experts recommend leaving the ice on for 10-15 minutes at a time. Ice is preferred over heat for treating injuries such as sprains, bruises, and torn muscles.

Beneficial supplementation:

Vitamin C:
Calcium:
DLPA (DL-Phenylalanine):
Herbs: Black Cohosh Root, Bugleweed, Catnip, Chaparral, Comfrey, Cornsilk, Fenugreek, Hops, Lady's Slipper, Mullein, Pau D' Arco, Valerian, White Willow Bark, Wild Yam (muscle pain). and Wintergreen.

PROSTATE TROUBLE

The prostate is a small donut-shaped organ which encircles the urethra at its junction with the bladder. The urethra is the tube that carries urine from the bladder to the end of the penis. When the prostate is enlarged, it narrows the urethra, blocking the passing of urine. Urinary problems and painful and urgent urination are common prostate disorders. Prostate troubles is one of the most common afflictions of men. Medical authorities estimate that over half of the men past age 45 suffer from prostate trouble. At age 80 or over, as many as 95 percent of men suffer prostate distress. Occurrence of prostate cancer is increasing.

Prostatitis is the inflammation of the prostate, a male sex gland. The usual cause of prostatitis in men in their 20s and 30s is a bacterial infection from another area of the body which has invaded the prostate. Symptoms of acute prostatitis are local pain, fever, frequent urination, inability to empty bladder fully, accompanied by a burning sensation, and blood or pus in the urine.

Prostatic enlargement (BHP or Benign Prostatic Hypertrophy) is the most common prostate problem. BHP is usually found in older males, and is often due to gradual enlargement over a period of several years. The prostate which is normally the size of a walnut can swell to the size of an orange. Symptoms of long-term prostatitis are frequent and burning urination, and lower back pain. As prostatitis becomes more advanced, urination becomes increasingly difficult. Prostate enlargement is quite common, especially for men past the age of 60.

What to do:

* Increase intake of foods which contain zinc (seafood, spinach, mushrooms, whole grains and sunflower seeds) and take a zinc supplement to relieve

painful symptoms and swelling.

* Add bee pollen to your diet which has provided substantial relief possibly due to its magnesium, zinc, unsaturated fatty acid, and sex hormone content.

* Increase fluid intake to meet increased needs during infection and to stimulate urine flow, thus preventing retention of urine.

* Take plenty of time to urinate until you are completely finished when nature calls, but do not strain. Several weeks of this training can strengthen bladder control.

* A well-balanced diet rich in fiber, non-citrus, alkaline-reacting food, vitamins A, the B complex and C, zinc, and essential fatty acids are important.

* Hot sitz baths and hot compresses can help relieve discomfort. Chamomile tea may be added to the water to help relieve pressure on the urethra and allow the bladder to empty fully.

* Alternate hot and cold sitz baths may be employed in chronic conditions and as maintenance therapy, once cure has been established.

* Avoid alcohol, caffeine, nicotine, and spicy foods which have negative irritating effects on the prostate.

* Avoid foods high in cholesterol, and foods containing saturated fat, hydrogenated oils or sugar. High serum levels of cholesterol have been associated with prostate disease.

Beneficial supplementation:

Vitamin A: 25,000 IU one to two times daily
B Complex: 50 mg three times daily
Vitamin B-6: 50-100 mg two times daily
Vitamin C: 1,000-2,000 mg thee times daily or more
Vitamin E: 400 IU two or three times daily
Calcium: 800-1,000 mg daily
Magnesium: 400-500 mg daily
Selenium: 100-300 mcg daily

Zinc: 50-100 mg daily (at this high dose you may also need to supplement 3-5 mg copper per day to maintain proper zinc-copper ratio.
Unsaturated fatty acids:
Protein:
Water:
Pumpkin seeds: up to 1/4 lb. daily
Bee pollen:
Lecithin:
Flax seed oil: 6-10 grams daily
Raw prostate tablets:
Herbs: Cayenne (Capsicum), False Unicorn Root, Goldenseal, Juniper Berries, Saw Palmetto Berries (oil extract), Siberian Ginseng, and Uva Ursi.

How to avoid:

Avoid foods high in cholesterol.

Eat a diet high in green and yellow vegetables. A 10-year study covering 122,261 men aged 40 and over showed that men with a low intake of green and yellow vegetables suffered prostate cancer twice as much as those men who ate plenty of vegetables. Scientists speculate that green and yellow vegetables are rich in vitamin A which may be responsible for the lower rate of prostate cancer.

PSORIASIS

Psoriasis, a recurring disease, is characterized by eruptions on the skin of red circular patches of all sizes covered with dry silvery scales. The patches enlarge slowly forming more extensive patches. Psoriasis mainly appears on the knees and legs, elbows and arms, scalp, ears, and lower back. The symptoms tend to flare up acutely with remissions.

It appears that psoriasis may result from faulty nutrition and faulty utilization of fats. Stress, constipation, excess meat eating (taurine), possible copper excess/zinc deficiency, food allergies, liver or kidney malfunctions, candida overgrowth, previous immunization, and acid/alkaline imbalance may also play a role in flareups.

Psoriasis has been considered practically incurable by orthodox methods.

What to do:

* Exposure to sunlight or ultraviolet light reduces the scaling and redness.

* Reduce animal protein and animal fat.

* Vitamin E (internal and external) is beneficial for lesions.

* Keep the skin clean to prevent infection.

* Castor oil packs applied to lower abdomen for 45 minutes to 1 and 1/2 hours nightly.

* Lightly brush off scales with loofah brush. Then apply liquid comfrey over the lesions. This can help reduce redness and scaling and in some cases, clearing of skin in some areas.

* Milk Thistle (Silymarin) is excellent for liver cleansing. Liver malfunction may be largely responsible for psoriasis. Both organs (the liver and the skin) are largely responsible for toxin removal of the body.

249

Beneficial supplementation:

Vitamin A: 50,000-100,000 IU daily during the first
week; reduce to 25,000 IU daily for three months.
Repeat.

B Complex: 100 mg twice daily

Vitamin B-6: 100-200 mg daily

Folic Acid: 25-75 mg daily

Vitamin C: 1,000-2,000 two to three times daily

Vitamin D:

Vitamin E: 1,500 IU

Bioflavonoids:

Magnesium:

Sulphur: (ointment)

Zinc: 25-50 mg three times daily (If bowel upset
occurs, reduce dosage.)

Lecithin: three tbsp daily

Essential Fatty Acids: i.e. Flax seed oil

Herbs: Burdock Root, Chickweed, Common Figwart,
Mullein, Slippery Elm (tea), and Yellow American
Saffron (tea).

SCURVY

Scurvy is a condition that is caused by a lack of vitamin C in the diet. It is characterized by weakness, anemia, loss of appetite, edema, spongy gums, loose teeth, hard bumps of the muscles of the legs. There is increased risk of infection and eventual breakdown of collagen.

Most animals synthesize their own vitamin C, but man, apes, and guinea pigs must rely upon dietary sources.

The Recommended Daily Allowance for vitamin C is 45 milligrams. According to Dr. Linus Pauling, Ph.D., who is probably the world's foremost authority on vitamin C, as well as other authorities, the RDAs provide insight as to the minimal amount needed daily to prevent deficiency disease, they are in no way amounts recommended to maintain optimal levels of health.

According to Pauling, to our surprise many Americans may be suffering from borderline scurvy. Large groups of people have increased need for vitamin C, including smokers, drinkers, the elderly, expecting or lactating mothers, athletes, and individuals under stress.

For example, each cigarette an individual smokes destroys 25 mg of vitamin C. Research shows that on the average, cigarette smokers have a 20 percent lower dietary intake of vitamin C than non-smokers. Blood serum levels of vitamin C in smokers is on average 25-40 percent lower than non-smokers. It is estimated that an additional vitamin C intake of a minimum of 133 mg per day would be necessary to raise smokers' serum levels to the levels in non-smokers.

Taking vitamin supplements protected both smokers and non-smokers against low serum vitamin C levels. Among non-smokers, a 3.5 percent of supplement users and 14.5 percent of non-users had low vitamin C levels. Among smokers, 9.8 percent of supplement users and 35.7 percent of non-users had low vitamin C levels.

What to do:

A deficiency of vitamin C is usually fairly easy to remedy. Increase your intake of vitamin C.

A number of supplements are available which provide vitamin C including Ascorbic Acid, Calcium Ascorbate, Sodium Ascorbate, Acerola Cherries, Bioflavonoids, Hesperidin, Rutin, Rose Hips, etc.

Ascorbic Acid: Synthetic high potency form of vitamin C.

Calcium Ascorbate: Synthetic high potency non-acidic form of vitamin C.

Sodium Ascorbate: Synthetic high potency form of vitamin C.

Acerola Cherries: Natural low potency source of vitamin C. Sometimes called Acerola C.

Bioflavonoids, Hesperidin, Rutin, and Rose Hips: Natural low potency forms of vitamin C which contain bioflavonoids and other enzymes which help C assimilate. Rose hips are the richest natural source of vitamin C.

Foods high in vitamin C include: Citrus fruits, berries, green and leafy vegetables, tomatoes, cauliflower, potatoes, and sweet potatoes. Fresh, raw foods will contain highest amounts of vitamin C. Methods of preparation destroy varying amounts of vitamin C.

Before fresh vegetables are eaten or cooked, they should be washed so that chemical sprays and dirt are removed. Soaking should be avoided because water soluble nutrients such as vitamin C can leach out.

Vegetable skins should be left on or pared as thinly as possible to retain nutrients.

Cooking time should be kept to the absolute minimum to retain all nutrients. Vitamin C is easily destroyed by cooking. Steaming will retain more nutrient content in comparison to boiling. At least half of the nutrients will be retained by steaming that would have been lost by boiling. Baked vegetables (like baked potatoes) will also have a higher concentration of nutrients than boiled vegetables. However, vegetables baked in juices (roasting) will lose more of some vitamins than if boiled.

Foods high in vitamin C content:

Black currants (1 cup)	202 mgs vitamin C
Papaya (1)	187 mgs vitamin C
Guava (1)	165 mgs vitamin C
Orange juice (1 cup)	124 mgs vitamin C
Melon-cantaloupe (1/2)	112 mgs vitamin C
Grapefruit juice (1 cup)	94 mgs vitamin C
Kohlrabi (1 cup)	87 mgs vitamin C
Strawberries (1 cup)	85 mgs vitamin C
Broccoli (1 cup)	82 mgs vitamin C
Kale (1 cup)	80 mgs vitamin C
Kiwi(1)	75 mgs vitamin C
Brussels sprouts (1 cup)	74 mgs vitamin C
Cauliflower (1 cup)	71 mgs vitamin C
Orange (1)	70 mgs vitamin C
Peppers-sweet (1/2 cup)	62 mgs vitamin C
Rutabaga (1 cup)	60 mgs vitamin C
Elderberries (1 cup)	52 mgs vitamin C
Asparagus (1 cup)	44 mgs vitamin C
Gooseberries (1 cup)	42 mgs vitamin C
Grapefruit (1/2)	42 mgs vitamin C
Potatoes (1 flesh and skin)	30 ms vitamin C
Sweet potato (1)	30 mgs vitamin C

Beneficial supplementation:

Calcium Ascorbate:
Ascorbic Acid:
Acerola Cherries:
Bioflavonoids:
Hesperidin:
Rutin:
Rose Hips:

Did You Know...

You can get food poisoning from your pet turtle? Pet turtles can be hazardous to their owners health because they are often carriers of salmonella bacteria.

SKIN CANCER

About 90 percent of all cases of skin cancer (malignant melanoma) are thought to be due to sun exposure. The incidence of skin cancer in the United States has risen 1,500 percent over the past 50 years. About 27,000 Americans will develop melanoma this year and 6,300 will die from it. The risk of developing melanoma is about one in 120. Young children and teenagers are at the greatest risk.

Malignant melanoma is a deadly skin cancer that is killing 30 percent more Americans today than it did less than 20 years ago. The reasons are:
* The growing intensity of sunlight because of the depletion of the earth's ozone layer.
* Trends in swimwear to expose more skin.

Anyone can develop skin cancer, but having three of the following risk factors increases your chance of developing melanoma by three to four times. Having four or more of these factors carries a 25 fold greater risk. They are:
* **Being a blond or redhead.**
* **Having blue or green eyes.**
* **Having abundant freckles on the upper back.**
* **Having fair skin that burns or freckles lately**
* **Having a tendency to develop a red, bumpy rash after exposure to the sun.**
* **Having a relative who has developed melanoma.**
* **Having at least three blistering sunburns before the age of 20.**
* **Working outdoors for three or more summers as a teenager.**

Individuals with two or more risk factors should be alert to the first signs of melanoma because when caught early the cancer is curable. It is almost always fatal after small black or blue tumors appear on the skin. An early melanoma lesion can resemble an ordinary mole with irregular edges, a red scaly patch or a pale waxy nodule.

Approximately 80 percent of skin cancers are found in the head and neck area. Other vulnerable areas include other highly exposed areas such as the hands and forearms.

Skin cancer is not the only consequence of sun exposure. Premature aging (wrinkles, dry skin, age spots and moles, etc.) may not be as dangerous as skin cancer, but much time, energy and money are often spent in futile attempts to undue the consequences.

Of all the factors which effect your skin, age, heredity, eating and drinking habits, smoking, stress, health, rest and exercise, your degree of sun exposure and how you protect your skin when you are outdoors is one of the most significant factors which determines the youthful look and feel of your skin.

Sunshine is the most harmful influence there is for your skin. Years of exposure to the sun exaggerates and accelerates one's natural aging process. It is the primary cause of premature aging; causing wrinkling, thinning of the skin, and the appearance of broken blood vessels and brownish discolorations known as "age spots." Sunshine accelerates the normal loss of moisture, and elasticity of the skin. Twenty years of sunning can leave you looking 15 to 20 years older than you really are.

You can easily check your own skin to prove this. There is one area on your body which has probably seen little sunlight in comparison to the rest of you, your buttocks or breasts. Look carefully at the skin of your face, arms, neck and upper chest and compare it to the skin of your buttocks and breasts. Look for age spots, wrinkling, "broken" blood vessels, smoothness, a leather-like look and feel, discoloration and other signs of aging. You will probably be surprised that your buttocks look much more youthful than the skin on the other areas of your body. If the sun was not the cause of the aging on the exposed skin, then wouldn't all the skin age evenly, regardless of its amount of sun-exposure?

Many of you have experienced sunburn, which is not only extremely painful, is extremely damaging to your skin. Individual episodes of sunburn, particularly during childhood and adolescence, have been linked to the development of skin cancer which is potentially life threatening and can be extremely disfiguring.

A suntan, as well as a sunburn, is damaging to the skin. The ultra-violet rays of the sun penetrate through the skin which responds by producing and redistributing melanin pigment in order to minimize damage to itself. In other words, the tan is an attempt to protect the skin from further damage. The darker the tan, the deeper the damage. Even after the tan fades, the damage remains and accumulates over the years. This is the reason it takes years to start seeing the harmful effects.

How to avoid:

Fortunately, there are a large number of sunscreens available we can take advantage of. Today sunscreens are available in a wide range of sun protection factors which you can and should use according to your degree of sensitivity.

Fair skinned individuals should choose a higher sun protection factor because they have less melanin pigment which provides natural protection. Without natural protection, fair skinned individuals are the most sensitive to the damaging ultra-violet rays of the sun and therefore require the most protection. Fair skinned individuals are also more susceptible to wrinkles.

Darker skinned individuals have higher amounts of naturally occurring melanin pigment and do not seem to be as sensitive. None-the-less, it is still very important that they use sunscreen if they want to keep their skin beautiful, prevent premature wrinkles and age spots.

The American Cancer Society, the Skin Cancer Foundation, and the American Academy of Dermatology recommend these precautions:

* Avoid sun exposure between 10 a.m. and 3 p.m. when ultra-violet rays are most intense.

* Wear a hat, tightly woven protective clothing, and sunglasses (make sure they protect from UV rays) when exposed to the sun. **NOTE:** Sunglasses with lens which do not provide protection from UV rays are very dangerous. Regular tinted lens provide an illusion to your eyes that it

is darker than it is and your pupils will dilate (like in a dark room) making your eyes extremely sensitive to damage.

    * Before sun exposure, apply a sun screen with a Sun Protection Factor of 15 or more. **NOTE:** Remember to reapply your sun screen if you are in extremely hot weather or are involved in activity causing you to perspire. If you are in or around water, the sun's rays are actually more intense because they are reflected, therefore adequate protection is extremely important. You are not protected if you are underwater either, you need to wear a water-proof sun screen and reapply it often.

    Cloudy weather conditions can give one a false sense of security when you are outdoors. Most people think that a partly cloudy or foggy day means a day without sunburn. This is not true because as much as 80 percent of the ultra-violet rays of the sun can be transmitted through clouds and fog and can still cause a sunburn. Wind may also increase one's chances of overexposure to the sun because it may seem cooler allowing you to remain comfortably in the sun for longer periods.

    It is also important to use sun screen on your lips. Too much sun can cause cracking, peeling and blistering of the lips. Individuals who are sensitive to fever blisters on their lips also need to take special protective care of the rest of their body.

SKIN PROBLEMS

The skin is an organ and has functions just like the liver or stomach. The skin protects, secretes, and absorbs. It is a major part of the excretory system responsible for waste removal. In fact, the skin is actually the largest organ in the body.

The skin is made up of two major parts: the outer surface called the epidermis, and the inner layer called the dermis.

The epidermis is the layer which you see and touch. The function of this layer is to protect the layers of skin underneath. The outermost layer (stratum corneum) of skin cells are actually dead. These cells are continuously shed and then replaced.

The epidermal layers below the stratum corneum are the stratum lucidum, the stratum granulosum, and stratum germinativum. The single layer of cells in the stratum germinativum (called the stratum basale) is capable of continual cell reproduction. As these cells multiply, they are pushed up toward the surface and eventually are shed from the top layer of the epidermis, the stratum corneum.

The inner layer of skin is called the dermis. This layer serves as the foundation for the outer surface. It is made up of living cells, consisting largely of connective tissue. It also contains numerous blood vessels, nerves, glands, and hair follicles are also embedded in the dermis. The function of the inner layer is to provide water and nutrients to the entire skin.

Connective tissue is a thick net of insoluble protein fibers. The network of these protein fibers, a supporting structure, is largely made from two main types of proteins: Collagen and elastin. Within connective tissue, collagen gives structure, and elastin gives flexibility to the tissue.

In addition to the inner layer of skin, we also have connective tissue in the nails, hair, tendons, ligaments, cartilage and in the matrix of the bone. The bone matrix is made almost entirely of collagen, 96 percent. There is also connective tissue in the arteries, and especially the arteries coming from the heart, such as the aorta.

Common problems include:

Boils (or furuncles) are infected nodules on the skin with a central core of pus surrounded by inflamed and swollen tissue. A boil forms when the skin tissue is weakened by chafing, lowered resistance due to disease, or inadequate nutrition. Boil symptoms include itching, mild pain, and localized swelling. Proper hygiene is essential for treatment. Infected areas should be washed several times a day and swabbed with antiseptic. Vitamins A and C, and zinc are important for healing and prevention.

Dry skin can result from a deficiency of vitamins A, C, or B Complex. Because the oils of the skin are largely unsaturated, the unsaturated fatty acids are needed for moist skin. Dry skin is more common as we increase in age because Na-PCA, the skin's natural moisturizer, decreases with age. Vitamins A, B complex and Vitamin C, Unsaturated fatty acids (Cod Liver Oil, Flax Seed Oil, Evening Primrose Oil, etc.), and Na-PCA (cream or spray) can help relieve dry skin. **(see section on Dry Skin)**

Fungus infestations include athlete's foot, ringworm, infestations on or around the genitals and anus or around the mouth (causing thrush), or inflammations on the fingers or under the fingernails. The most common causes of these infestations is the destruction of beneficial bacteria by antibiotics, drugs, or radiation, resulting in undesirable fungi. Vitamins A, B Complex and C, raw fruits, vegetables, whole grains, yogurt and especially acidophilus are important for recovery.

Itching skin often rises from an iron deficiency, especially if there is no other diseases present. Numbness and tingling sometimes accompany the itching signaling slight nerve dysfunction. Itching may also accompany rashes and hives which may be caused from allergies or chemical sensitivities and stress. **(See section on Itching)**

Lip problems including sore lips, whistle marks, and cracks at the corners of the mouth, usually indicate a vitamin B complex deficiency (especially B-2, B-6, folic acid and pantothenic acid). Unsaturated fatty acids also may be lacking. Supplements of these nutrients often readily clears up the problem. Remember to wear sunscreen on your lips when outdoors.

Oily skin (and hair) has been produced in persons only slightly deficient in vitamin B-2. Doses of 15 milligrams daily have cleared up the condition. The entire B Complex may be helpful.

Prickly heat is a rash consisting of tiny pimples that itch, sometimes quite severely. The rash is usually caused by inadequate function of the sweat glands of the body. This is often due to stress and fatigue. Vitamin C (1-5 grams daily) is often very beneficial combined with good nutrition and adequate rest. Cornstarch may also help when sprinkled on areas susceptible to breakouts (inbetween thighs, behind knees and inside elbow, etc.)

Rashes are commonly associated with allergies, chemical sensitivities, and heavy metal toxicity. Stress can make rashes (as well as other skin conditions) worse. The skin is the largest organ of elimination and can throw off toxins and poisons. Inner cleansing and skin brushing opens pores and eliminates dead wastes. Alfalfa and other blood purifiers, and vitamin C (3-6 grams daily) have been very beneficial for many people.

Scars and stretch marks may be prevented and removed by vitamin E (400-800 IU) taken internally and applied externally daily.

Sunburn can be relieved by applying aloe vera gel. In addition take B Complex vitamins, PABA, vitamins C and E, calcium and zinc. **(See section on Skin Cancer)**

Warts are commonly of viral origin and occur when the body's immune system is low. 25,000-50,000 IU of vitamin A have caused warts to disappear. Vitamin E (400-800 IU) taken orally and applied topically is also beneficial.

Wrinkles and the loss of elasticity result from a damaged mechanism called cross-linking, in which proteins are bonded together, preventing them from

261

functioning properly. Sunlight, alcohol and tobacco are major offenders. Cross-linking can be slowed down or prevented by avoiding these and by taking antioxidants such as vitamins A, B-1, C, E, and zinc and selenium.

Beneficial supplementation:

Vitamin A:
B Complex:
Vitamin B-1:
Vitamin B-2:
Vitamin B-6:
Niacin:
Vitamin C:
Vitamin D:
Vitamin E:
Selenium:
Silica:
Zinc:
Cysteine: Take in one to three ratio with Vitamin C
    (i.e., 1,000 mg Cysteine: 3,000 mg Vitamin C).
Cod Liver Oil:
Flax Seed Oil:
Herbs: Alfalfa, Aloe Vera, Burdock, Comfrey,
    Dandelion, Goldenseal, Horsetail, Oatstraw,
    Queen of the Meadow, Yarrow, Yellow Dock.

How to avoid:

There are many different nutrients involved in the general maintenance and health of connective tissue. One of the most important of these nutrients may be silica. Silica is clearly one of the most effective components in connective tissue. Because silica is so abundantly found in nature, we seem to tend to forget that we may become deficient in it. But due to the great amount of processing of our foods, much of it is lost.

Silica plays an important role in the degree of elasticity of the elastin tissue. Silica has been shown to thicken and preserve elasticity. Silica also has a role in "cementing" the skin together and also in "holding" calcium in the bone. It has been shown that in conditions such as osteoporosis, silica is actually lost from the bone before calcium is. The reverse is also true that bone can be re-mineralized by the addition of silica.

Vitamin C is also important for the integrity of connective tissue because it is needed for collagen formation. Vitamin C acts as a glue that holds tissue together. In addition, vitamin C has the ability to double the healing rate of cuts and wounds and is a powerful antioxidant that helps prevent cross-linking of the skin that contributes to premature wrinkling.

Other important nutrients include manganese, magnesium, iron, vitamins B-5 and B-6. Also important are two amino acids which are known to be good sulfur-donators which seems to be important for the formation of chondroitin sulphate. This is a principal component for the intracellular substance of connective tissue. These amino acids are L-taurine and L-cysteine.

Supplements are a very important part of health and skin care today. For a number of reasons, our foods do not contain the nutrient levels that they did years ago. Stress, smoking, alcoholic beverages, sunshine, pollution, soil depletion, and the aging factor itself, increase our need for certain vitamins, minerals, antioxidants and other nutrients.

Supplements such as vitamins, minerals, amino acids, antioxidants, etc. can greatly enhance one's health and therefore one's skin.

SMOKING

Smoking is the addictive habit of smoking cigarettes for physical and psychological causes. Smokers commonly experience pallor, premature aging, discolored teeth and skin, bad breath, coated tongue, frequent colds, bronchitis, emphysema, and lung cancer.

Peer pressure has created most smokers, along with the industry's advertising. Nicotine is a highly addictive drug and has real physical dependence. In addition, smoking is easily associated with positive actions which makes quitting a very difficult task.

Smoking is a causative factor in many diseases, reducing not only the length of life, but also the quality. Smokers have more colds, sinusitis, bronchitis, emphysema, heart attacks, strokes and other upper respiratory and circulatory problems than non-smokers. Smoking aggravates diabetes, ulcers, high blood pressure, Burger's disease, and glaucoma, and may cause osteoporosis, smaller babies, miscarriages, stillbirths, and lung cancer.

What to do:

* Vitamin C (5-15 grams daily) supplementation is of critical importance for smokers. Each cigarette destroys 25 mg of vitamin C in the body. At one pack a day, this far exceeds the normal intake of this vitamin. Prolonged deficiency of vitamin C may be a factor in the increase in cancer in heavy smokers. Vitamin C also helps detoxify nicotine.

* Vitamin E supplementation is also important for smokers. The carbon monoxide in the smoke destroys the oxygen-carrying ability of the hemoglobin in the blood.

* Quit smoking or cut down the amount that you smoke. The moment you quit smoking your body starts to recover.

265

Suggestions for cutting down on cigarette smoking:

* Smoke only half of each cigarette.
* Each day, postpone lighting your first cigarette one hour.
* Decide that you will smoke only during odd or even hours of the day.
* Decide beforehand how many cigarettes you will smoke during the day. For each additional smoke, donate a dollar to your favorite charity.
* Do not buy cigarettes by the carton. Wait until one pack is empty before buying another.
* Stop carrying cigarettes with you at home and work. Make them difficult to get to.
* Make yourself aware of each cigarette by using the opposite hand or putting cigarettes in an unfamiliar location.
* Do not smoke "automatically." Smoke only those you really want.
* Reward yourself in some other way than smoking.
* Reach for a glass of juice, piece of fruit or raw vegetable instead of a cigarette.
* Change your eating habits to aid in cutting down. For example, drink milk, which is frequently considered incompatible with smoking.
* Do not empty your ashtrays. This will not only remind you of how many cigarettes you have had, but also the smell of stale butts will be unpleasant.

Beneficial supplementation:

Beta Carotene: 25,000 IU one to three times daily
B Complex: (extra B-1)
Niacin: 100-1,000 mg two times daily
Vitamin C: 5-15 grams daily
Vitamin E:
Selenium:
Zinc:
Herbs: Hops, Skullcap, Valerian, Catnip, Slippery Elm.

How to avoid:

Instead of smoking after meals, get up from the table and brush your teeth or go for a walk.

If you always smoke while driving, take public transportation.

You may need to temporarily avoid situations you strongly associate with the pleasurable aspects of smoking such as watching your favorite TV show, sitting in your favorite chair, having a cocktail before dinner.

Develop a clean non-smoking environment around yourself-at home and at work.

Until you are confident of your ability to stay off cigarettes, limit your socializing to healthful, outdoor activities or situations where smoking is prohibited.

If you must be in a situation where you will be tempted to smoke (such as a cocktail or dinner party), try to associate with the non-smokers there.

Keep oral substitutes handy like carrots, celery, sunflower seeds, apples, raisins, sugarless gum, etc.

Take ten deep breaths and hold the last one while lighting a match. Exhale slowly and blow out the match. Pretend it is a cigarette and crush it out in an ashtray.

When you get the urge, if possible, take a shower or bath.

Learn to relax. Concentrate on a peaceful image, practice meditation or yoga.

Did You Know...

Chocolate is harmful to your pets?
Chocolate contains theobromine, a caffeine-related stimulant, that can lead to urinary incontinence, seizures and death in dogs and cats.

SNORING

Snoring is a noise made while sleeping due to vibration against the soft pallet located in the back of the mouth. Snoring usually only occurs when individuals are sleeping on their back.

Most people who snore are at least 20 percent over there ideal weight. The use of depressants including alcohol, antihistamines, sleeping pills and tranquilizers can induce snoring in many individuals. Also, physical conditions such as excess cartilage in the back of the mouth can cause one to snore.

What to do:

* Turn onto your side rather than your back. Prop pillows on either side of your body to prevent rolling over onto your back.

* Devise a means to avoid sleeping on your back. For example, a "snore ball" can be made by cutting a small solid rubber ball in half. Using two pieces of velcro, attach the flat side of the ball onto your pajamas. This should prevent you from sleeping on your back.

* Lose weight. Three out of four people who snore are overweight.

How to avoid:

Avoid alcoholic beverages within two hours of going to bed.

Avoid tranquilizers, sleeping pills, and antihistamines before bedtime.

Wear a cervical collar. It keeps the chin up and the windpipe open.

Tilt the head of the bed upwards. You may place six to eight inch wooden blocks under the front legs of the bed. Elevating the head will keep the airways open. **NOTE:** Using extra pillows is ineffective because the airways become kinked.

Maintain ideal weight.

STRESS

Stress is any kind of physical or emotional strain on the body or mind. Stress is with us all the time. It is an unavoidable part of our lives. Stress is unique and personal to each of us. What may be stressful to one person may actually be relaxing to another.

Physical stress occurs when an external or natural change or force acts upon the body. Extreme heat or cold, overwork, injuries, malnutrition, illness, and exposure to drugs or poisons, are examples of physical stress.

Emotional stress may be a result of fear, hate, love, anger, tension, grief, frustration, and/or anxiety. Too much emotional stress can cause the immune system to wear down and physical illness such as high blood pressure, ulcers, asthma, migraine headaches, strokes, cancer and heart disease can occur.

Emotional and physical stresses also may be combined in special body conditions such as pregnancy, adolescence and aging. During these times, body metabolism is increased or lowered, changing the body's physical functions, which, in turn, affect a person's mental and emotional outlook on life.

A certain amount of stress may be useful as a motivational factor, but too much of the wrong kind of stress can be detrimental. Recognizing early signs of stress and then doing something about it can make an important difference in the quality of life.

Physiologically, stress causes an increase in the production of adrenal hormones which increases the metabolism of proteins, fats, and carbohydrates, producing instant energy for the body to use. As a result, there is also an increased excretion of protein, potassium, and phosphorus and a decreased storage of calcium. Many of the disorders related to stress are not a direct result of stress but a result of nutrient deficiencies caused by increased metabolic rate during stress. Vitamin C is utilized by the adrenal glands during stress and any stress which is sufficiently severe or prolonged will cause a depletion of vitamin C in the tissues.

What to do:

* Physical exercise is one of the most effective means of relieving emotional stress.
* Relax. Get away from the situation and take several deep breaths. Find activities that give you pleasure and are good for your physical and mental well-being, such as golf, walking, fishing, biking, music, reading, playing with a pet or children, etc.
* Mentally think of something that produces an inner smile or glow. Thinking of an adored person, an amusing situation, your pet or some other "melt moment" induces calmness, reduces heart rate, relaxes muscle tension and gives a sense of well-being.
* Do not keep things bottled up inside. If something is bothering you, let it out. Talking to someone can help relieve stress and make you feel better. Keeping a journal and writing letters can also help you get things off your chest and relieve stress.
* Crying can be a healthy way to bring relief to anxiety, and it might even prevent a headache or other physical consequence.
* Avoid drugs. Drugs are habit forming and create more stress than they take away.
* Chocolate may not be all bad! Chocolate contains high amounts of pyrazines which stimulate the pleasure center in the brain. This interrupts stress signals and helps cheer you up. The sugar in chocolate also raises the level of brain serotonin, a natural chemical that soothes frazzled nerves. **NOTE:** Sugar does have a great number of detriments and should almost always be avoided, especially by sugar sensitive individuals, such as hypoglycemics. Chocolate treats also often contain saturated fats and/or hydrogenated oils which should be consumed in limited quantities.

* Replacement of lost nutrients such as B Complex (especially B-1, B-6, B-12, and pantothenic acid), vitamin C, magnesium, potassium, phosphorus, zinc, etc., is of critical importance to maintain health. When you do not provide the body with adequate and complete nutrition it is more difficult for the body to recover from the physical effects of stress.

* B Complex vitamins help maintain the health of the nervous system. Even a slight deficiency can cause irritability and depression.

* Vitamin B-1: Several dietary factors interfere with he ability of the body to utilize vitamin B-1 (thiamine). Tea (tannic acid), sugar, and alcohol consumption raise thiamine requirements in the body.

* Vitamin B-5 (Pantothenic acid) improves the ability of even well-nourished people to withstand stress.

* Inositol converts into tryptophan and then into serotonin in the brain which is crucial for sleep. Stress related insomnia may be associated with a deficiency in this B vitamin.

* Vitamin C: Physical and emotional stress can increase the need for vitamin C by 50 times. In addition, smoking (which often increases during stressful times) depletes the tissues of vitamin C.

* Magnesium is also drained from the body by stress. Studies indicate that a magnesium deficiency weakens the body's ability to cope with stress and makes one more sensitive to stimuli such as noise and bright lights, etc.

* GABA acts as an inhibitory neurotransmitter that prevents too many messages from being relayed across the brain.

Beneficial supplementation:

Vitamin A: 25,000-50,000 IU daily
B Complex: (extra B-1,B-5, B-6, and B-12) 50 mg two
   to three times daily
Inositol:
Vitamin C: To saturation level
Vitamin E: 400-800 IU daily
Calcium: 800-1,000 mg daily
Chromium:
Copper:
Iron:
Magnesium: 600-1,000 mg daily
Potassium: 250 mg daily
Phosphorus: 150 mg daily
Selenium:
Zinc: 25-50 mg one to two times daily
Methionine:
Essential Fatty Acids: (Flaxseed Oil, Evening Primrose
   Oil, GLA and EPA)
Raw Adrenal: one tablet three times daily
GABA:
Herbs: Alfalfa, Chamomile, Ginseng, Gotu Kola, Hops, Kelp,
   Lady's Slipper, Passion Flower, and Valerian.

How to avoid:

Make time for fun. Schedule time for recreation into your busy agenda. This gives you something to look forward to and a break from your daily routine is excellent for relaxation.

Make sure you get adequate rest and eat well. If you are irritable and tense from lack of sleep or not eating correctly, you are less able to deal with stress.

Avoid coffee and other stimulants.

Do not overburden yourself with work or situations. If you need help ask for it. If you simply do not have the time, say no when asked to take on additional responsibility.

Talk to someone about your worries and concerns before they get out of hand.

THYROID DISORDERS

The thyroid, located in the base of the neck, plays a key role in controlling the body's metabolic rate and glucose level. It is controlled by secretions from the pituitary and hypothalamus.

Basic thyroid disorders include hypothyroidism, hyperthyroidism and goiter.

Hypothyroidism: This is an endocrine mis-function involving an underactive thyroid due to atrophy. Possible causes include; iodine deficiency, deficiency of vitamins A, E, or zinc, enzyme deficiency, diet pills, or pituitary disorders.

Juvenile hypothyroidism is due to a deficiency of thyroid hormone during fetal or early development. Causes are inborn errors of iodine metabolism, abnormal development of the thyroid, interference of thyroid hormone production and dietary deficiency.

Symptoms include fatigue, headaches, chronic or recurrent infection, dry skin, eczema, psoriasis, acne, menstrual disorders, painful menstruation, depression, cold sensitivity, psychological problems. In addition, a high percentage of hypothyroid patients suffer from iron-deficiency anemia.

Hypothyroidism is often overlooked because of its wide variety of symptoms. Hypothyroidism is often confused with hypoglycemia because of the thyroid's association with blood sugar.

Hyperthyroidism: (Also called Graves' Disease) This involves excessive production of thyroid hormone with growth or atrophy of thyroid gland, increased metabolic rate, and possible bulging of eyes. Causes include deficiencies of vitamin A, E, or B-6, liver damage causing insufficient enzyme production, or diet pills.

Symptoms include insomnia, nervousness, weakness, perspiration, over-activity, sensitivity to heat, weight loss, and tremors. The heart, if the thyroid is overactive and enlarged, may suffer systolic hypertension and possible heart failure. The thyroid is usually enlarged or nodular.

Goiter: This is an enlargement of the thyroid gland due to iodine deficiency of natural goitrogen in foods such as cabbage or kale that block synthesis of thyroid hormone and therefore stimulate thyroid stimulating hormone (TSH) production.

* To determine the state of your thyroid a useful home test is the basal body temperature test as first suggested by Dr. Broda Barnes, M.D., Ph.D., one of the world's foremost authority on the thyroid gland. To do this, before rising in the morning, take your temperature by placing a thermometer under your armpit and leaving it there for ten minute. Do this for two or three days to get an average reading. Average ranges are 97.8 to 98.2 degrees F. Temperatures below this range suggest hypothyroidism, and those above this range suggest hyperthyroidism. Women should take their temperature on days 2 and 3 of the menstrual flow to get an accurate measurement.

What to do:

* The most common and effective treatment for thyroid disorders is supplementation of raw desiccated thyroid.
* Eat foods high in iodine, vitamins A, B Complex, C, and E, preferably raw.
Foods of usefulness include:

Brewer's yeast
Egg yolks
Garlic
Kelp, dulse
Mushrooms
Radishes
Seafood
Seaweed
Watercress
Wheat germ

* Vitamin A is commonly deficient because Hypothyroid individuals do not convert beta-carotene to vitamin A efficiently.

* Vitamin E increases iodine uptake by the thyroid and heals scars in the gland.

* Individuals who also have iron-deficiency anemia should eat a diet high in iron-rich foods and/or supplement iron.

Iron-rich foods include:

Liver
Fish
Fowl
Fruit
Green vegetables
Raisins
Brown rice

Beneficial supplementation:

Vitamin A: 10,000 IU one to three times daily (not beta carotene)

B Complex: 25-50 mg one to three times daily

Vitamin B-1: (for hyperthyroid individuals)

Vitamin B-2:

Vitamin B-3:

Vitamin B-6: (especially for hyperthyroid individuals) 50-100 mg one to two times daily

Vitamin C: 1,000+ mg three times daily

Vitamin E: 400-1,200 IU daily

Zinc: 25 mg two to three times daily

Copper: 1-3 mg daily

Essential Fatty Acids:

Kelp:

Tyrosine: (for hypothyroid)

Raw adrenal:

Raw thyroid:

Homeopathic thyroid dilutions:

How to avoid:

Avoid excessive or prolonged intake of diet pills or "speed."

Maintain a diet sufficient in the B Complex vitamins, vitamins C, A, E, iron, zinc, etc.

TONSILLITIS AND SORE THROAT

Tonsillitis is an inflammation of the tonsils, which are glands of the lymph tissue located on either side of the entrance to the throat. The tonsils and other lymphoid tissue are designed by nature to act as filtering agents for viruses, bacteria, and toxins. Not only do they protect us from external agents, they also act as sensitive barometers of our inner health. When the blood or lymph becomes overburdened with toxic waste or bacteria, these organs become inflamed and infected.

Tonsillitis may be caused by virus infections when the body's resistance is lowered or by an improper diet that is high in carbohydrates and low in protein and other nutrients. Constipation and allergies, particularly milk intolerance, are also commonly associated with tonsillitis.

Symptoms include pain, redness, and swelling in the back of the mouth, difficulty in swallowing, hoarseness and coughing. Headache, earache, fever and chills, nausea and vomiting, nasal obstruction and discharge, and enlarged lymph nodes throughout the body are additional possible symptoms.

What to do:

* Eat a diet high in fruits (except bananas) and vegetables.

* Avoid mucus forming foods (milk and dairy products).

* Drink lots of hot clear beverages-five to six cups a day. Red Raspberry, Sage, and Slippery Elm teas are all good for sore throat and tonsillitis.

* Drink lots of pineapple and citrus juices.

* Take vitamin C every hour until saturation level is reached. Then reduce dosage and take approximately every three hours.

* Change your toothbrush.
* Do not smoke and avoid smokers.
* The following gargles may be beneficial:

Vitamin C and Zinc :
Gargle with mouthwashes containing vitamin C
and/or zinc three to four times a day.

Lemon and salt:
Add one teaspoon salt and eight ounces lemon to
hot water. Gargle for five minutes at least three
times a day.

Goldenseal, Myrrh, and glycothymoline.:
Mix one ounce of the two herbs (as alcohol
tincture) with 16 ounces of glycothymoline.
Gargle four to six times daily.

Beneficial supplementation:

Vitamin A: (if acute)
Adults: 25,000 IU daily
Children: 10,000 IU three time daily
B Complex: 25-50 mg three times daily
Vitamin C: (if acute) 500-1,000 mg (chewable
preferred) every hour until saturation level is
reached.
For sore throat: 500-1,000 mg six times a day.
Vitamin D:
Vitamin E:
Zinc: 15-30 mg three times daily (lozenges preferred)
Protein:
Garlic: Two capsules three times a day.
Onion Syrup: One tsp three to six times daily.
Herbs: Echinacea, Bayberry Root, Ginger Root,
Goldenseal (gargle), Marigold Flowers (tincture as
throat swab), Pleurisy Root, and St. John's Wort.

How to avoid:

Change your toothbrush often.
Take vitamin C (3-5 grams, more if you smoke) every
day.

TOOTH DECAY

Tooth decay (cavities) is the primary dental problem in the United States. Most cavities are caused by persistent eating of refined sugars and starches, which mix with saliva to form an acid which erodes tooth enamel, and improper brushing.

Cavities, recognised as a small whole or darkening of the tooth enamel, in the early stages will usually involve no pain because there are no nerve endings close to the tooth surface.

Cavities in their later stages are enlarged and may be extremely painful.

What to do:

* Maintain proper dental hygiene; Brush, floss and rinse with mouthwash containing 3 percent hydrogen peroxide solution after each meal.
* Avoid refined sugars, starches and especially sticky sweets.
* See your dentist regularly for checkups and preventative care.

Beneficial supplementation:

Vitamin A:
B Complex:
Vitamin C:
Bioflavonoids:
Vitamin D:
Vitamin E:
Calcium:
Magnesium:
Potassium:

Silica:
Zinc:
Lysine:
Herbs: Horsetail, and Peppermint Oil (toothaches).

How to avoid:

One can control cavities by avoiding refined carbohydrate foods, eating a nutritionally balanced diet and properly cleansing the mouth, including brushing the teeth and gums and cleansing between the teeth with dental floss following meals and snacks.

Avoid simple carbohydrates, especially sticky sweets.

Avoid eating snacks between meals (especially raisins which stick to your teeth) unless you plan to brush immediately afterwards.

Certain kinds of cheese may help prevent tooth decay because they prevent acid from forming on teeth and promoting decay. The best cheeses are Swiss, cheddar, and monterrey jack.

Change your toothbrush about every month because bristles become worn and lose their effectiveness. In addition, toothbrushes are a perfect environment for heavy bacterial growth.

Professional cleaning and checkups are recommended once or twice a year.

Infants and children may benefit from fluorinated water and toothpaste, but numerous individuals oppose the use of fluoride because in high levels it is toxic. Studies claim fluoridated water is responsible for a 10-50 percent reduction in dental caries. Fluoride has no value for adult teeth. Fluoride is also associated with mottled (blotchy-discolored teeth) in children and adults.

Fluoride is especially detrimental for individuals who are:

Calcium deficient: Fluoride makes calcium reserves insoluble

Vitamin C deficient: Vitamin C is essential for calcium absorption.

Elderly:

Impaired in their renal functioning:

Diabetic: Prone to kidney disease

Arthritic:

Disturbed calcium metabolism:

Hyper or Hypothyroid: Fluoride is an iodine antagonist

Fluoride sensitive:

Pregnant:

Taking birth control pills:

Infants: Prone to abnormal bone development, depressed thyroid function, heart damage, and mottled teeth.

Did You Know...

Breast-fed babies are susceptible to a vitamin D deficiency?

Breast milk often contains inadequate quantities of vitamin D while regular milk and formula are fortified.

URINARY TRACT INFECTIONS

Urinary tract infections are inflammations of the bladder and/or urethra. About one-third of all women age 20 to 40 are likely to suffer from recurring urinary tract infections. Women get urinary infections 10 times more often than men.

Symptoms include:

Frequency and burning on urination.

Pain and tenderness over bladder area.

Intense desire to pass urine even after bladder has been emptied.

Possibly strong odored cloudy urine.

What to do:

Drink plenty of water 8 to 12 glasses a day. This encourages frequent urination which empties the bladder and flushes out bacteria. Dilating urine also eases urinary symptoms.

Make sure genital area is clean at all times. Proper hygiene is of critical importance.

Wear cotton underwear because they are more absorbent than nylon or synthetic underwear.

Drink cranberry juice: Drink at least three 6 ounce glasses per day. Cranberry juice has a high concentration of vitamin C. One cup of cranberry juice has over 100 mg. Vitamin C and can help kill E. coli, the most common cause of urinary tract infections. Cranberry juice also contains hippuric acid which tends to inhibit the growth of bacteria.

Beneficial supplementation:

Vitamin A: 10,000-25,000 IU two or more times daily for short periods.
Vitamin C: 2,000 mg three to six times daily, or to saturation.
Folic Acid: 40-80 mg daily
Pantothenic Acid: 100 mg twice daily
Niacin: 100 mg twice daily
Vitamin E: 400 IU one to two times daily
Acidophilus:
Cranberry juice: 3 or more 6 ounce glasses daily
Herbs: Barberry (uva ursi) tincture, Buchu, Couch Grass tincture, Echinacea, Garlic, Goldenseal tea, Juniper Berries, Parsley Root and Seed tea or tincture.

How to avoid:

Drink 8-12 glasses of water a day.
Use tampons instead of sanitary napkins. Bacteria can more easily build up on napkins.
Take showers instead of baths. Bacteria can easily travel up the urinary tract while you are sitting in the tub.
Do not use bubble bath, it can be irritating.
Avoid wearing tight jeans or slacks.
Wear cotton underwear.
Maintain proper hygiene, especially genital area.

VARICOSE VEINS

Varicose veins are veins that have become abnormally enlarged, twisted and swollen. They may occur any where, but are most commonly found in the legs.

Factors which may contribute to development of varicose veins are obesity, heredity, tight clothing, sedentary lifestyle, crossing the legs, pregnancy and nutritional deficiencies (vitamins E and C).

Symptoms include muscle cramps, fatigue of leg muscles, ankle swelling, eczema, and ulcers.

What to do:

* Elevating the legs while resting can help
* Regular use of a slant board can help.
* Application of topical white oak bark (i.e. oak bark poultice or salve) has proven to be helpful against varicose veins. It helps to strengthen the veins.
* Kelp also helps strengthen the veins.
* Adequate amounts of the B vitamins and vitamin C are necessary for the maintenance of strong blood vessels.
* Vitamin E, which can dilate blood vessels and improve circulation, can help prevent varicose veins.
* Avoid refined carbohydrates.
* Avoid wearing high heeled shoes which add additional stress.

Beneficial supplementation:

B Complex:
Vitamin C: 1,000+ mg three to four times daily
Bioflavonoids (rutin):
Vitamin E: 600-1,000 IU
Calcium:
Magnesium:
Manganese:

Selenium:
Silica:
Zinc:
Protein:
Unsaturated fatty acids:
Lecithin:
Black strap molasses:
Liquid chlorophyll:
Herbs: Butcher's Broom, Capsicum, Goldenseal,
    Horsetail, Kelp, Oatstraw, Parsley, White Oak
    Bark, Witch Hazel.

How to avoid:

Maintain adequate amounts of the B vitamins,
vitamins C and E.

WARTS

Warts are viral infections. The most common types are common, venereal and plantar warts. The symptoms are raised, irregular (common, venereal), or flat (plantar) growths on the skin. They may be symptomless or cause pain and discomfort.

Causes are a lowered resistance to the viral infection, and vitamin A deficiency due to improper diet. Deficiencies of vitamin A and zinc have also been associated with increased incidence of viral infections.

What to do:

* Apply vitamin E (28,000 IU) one or two times daily to help them go away. In addition, take 400-800 IU vitamin E orally.

* Make a paste with apple cider vinegar and Capsicum, put on wart and cover with bandage.

* Apply Tea Tree Oil.

* Make a paste with castor oil and baking soda and apply to wart each night. Cover with a bandage. Do not pick at the wart during the day, but allow three to six weeks for it to slough off.

Beneficial supplementation:

Vitamin A: (emulsified) 50,000 IU daily for six weeks
B Complex: 25-50 mg two to three times daily
Vitamin C: 3,000 mg to 8,000 daily
Bioflavonoids:
Vitamin E:
  Internally: 400-800 IU daily
  Externally: 28,000 IU twice daily
Zinc: 50-100 mg daily
Herbs: Aloe Vera, Black Walnut (externally), Garlic,
  Goldenseal, and Tea Tree Oil (externally).

WORMS
(Intestinal Parasites)

There are several types of parasites which can live in the human intestine, most commonly are pinworms, tapeworms, hookworms, roundworms and various protozoa. Parasites live upon or in another living organism at whose expense it obtains advantages (i.e. food and shelter).

Parasites irritate the intestinal lining and cause poor absorption of nutrients. Initially, most people have no symptoms and do not realize they have worms. As infection becomes worse, signs of worms include diarrhea, gas, weakness, fatigue, hunger pains, lactose intolerance, appetite loss, weight loss, irritation of anal area, and anemia.

No one is free from the risk of parasite infection although individuals with decreased immunity are more likely to suffer ill effects.

Foreign travel dramatically increases one's chances of becoming infected, although many individuals can become infected without even leaving the country.

Eating exotic dishes such as sushi (raw fish), carpaccio (raw meat), and steak tartare, greatly increases the likelihood of infection.

Microwave cooking increases the likelihood of getting parasites because these foods, especially meats, are often not thoroughly cooked.

Pets can also transmit parasites to humans. (All puppies are born with round worms.)

Children are often carriers. Parents and caretakers can get parasite eggs under their fingernails while changing diapers and pass along eggs to other children or to other family members.

Contaminated drinking water is perhaps the most common parasitic vehicle today. The protozoa Giardia lamblia is the most popular water-borne parasite in the country and has become a recognised problem. Research has shown Giardia is often related to chronic fatigue syndrome, allergies and ulcers.

Sexual contact, and especially anal sex, is another means of parasite transmittal.

Other etiologic considerations include: Poor diet (sugar and refined carbohydrates, excess dairy, excess acidity, excess meat, deficiency of raw green vegetables, excess cooked foods), constipation, poor hygiene, and upset internal ecology.

What to do:

* Personal hygiene is the most important factor for the control of pinworms.

* Insert a fresh garlic clove rectally at night. Garlic is antiparasitic, antiviral, and antifungal.

* Increase dietary intake of fresh garlic and supplement garlic as well.

* Black Walnut and Pink Root are antiparasitic and antifungal.

* Grapefruit Seed Extract, a protozoa-eliminating botanical compound, is antibacterial and antifungal.

* Cranberry Concentrate, which is very rich in digestive acids, has the ability to digest protein-like substances and provide an acid-like medium which helps to eradicate protozoa in the intestines.

* Sufficient stomach acid will destroy parasites contained in foods. Supplement hydrochloric acid.

* Avoid milk and dairy products.

* Avoid sugar and refined carbohydrates. Parasites thrive on simple sugars.

* Eat a moderate protein diet with only complex carbohydrates.

* Cleanse the gastrointestinal tract with natural bulking agents such as fiber and activated charcoal which has an inordinate capacity to absorb a variety of intestinal toxins, bacteria, and parasitic by-products.

* Following cleansing, the intestinal tract needs to be repopulated with milk-free acidophilus.

* Constipation, if present, must be overcome because worms will thrive if the bowels do not move loosely.

* A highly alkaline environment in the intestinal tract and colon will destroy parasites. Increase intake of alkaline forming foods such as:

Almonds
Apricots (especially dried)
Cabbage and raw greens
Carrots
Figs (especially dried)
Garlic and onion
Lima beans (dried)
Lemon
Pumpkin seeds (and pumpkin seed tea)

Beneficial supplementation:

Vitamin A:
B Complex:
Vitamin D:
Vitamin K:
Calcium:
Iron:
Sulfur (ointment form):
Protein:
Unsaturated fatty acids:
Hydrochloric acid:
Milk-free Acidophilus:
Pancreatic enzymes:
Herbs: Black Walnut, Blessed Thistle, Cranberry Concentrate, Garlic, Grapefruit Seed Extract, Pink Root, Senna, and Slippery Elm.

How to avoid:

In general, proper nutrition, proper disposal of human feces, good hygiene, proper washing and cooking of foods are required to avoid parasites.

Always wash your hands and scrub under the fingernails before eating, and especially after going to the bathroom.

A high fiber alkaline diet is the best prevention of infestation, and cure.

Avoid all raw, rare, or undercooked meats, fish and pork.

When eating out, avoid salad bars and make sure that most of the foods you choose are cooked thoroughly, especially fish.

Drink only filtered or bottled water.

Wear gloves when gardening and when cleaning and changing kitty litter.

Deworm your pets on a regular basis. Do not allow your pets to defecate in public areas, especially where children play.

YEAST INFECTION
(Candida Albicans)

Yeast infection is a local or systemic colonization of the skin or mucous membranes of the yeast Candida albicans, also called thrush.

Candida albicans is normally found in the mouth, digestive tract, vagina and skin of healthy people. Under normal conditions, the body's defense barriers and immune system keeps this fungus controlled and in limited existence. However, if the body's defenses are weakened by an improper diet, or if the general or local ecology of the body or tissues is severely altered, such as occurs with antibiotic use, Candida begin to flourish. As the yeast takes hold, it produces local irritation and sends systemic toxins throughout the body causing a number of symptoms: Fatigue, depression, constipation or diarrhea, gas, bloating, abdominal pain, muscle or joint pain, headaches, allergies, rashes, nail fungus, hypoglycemia, etc.

Vaginal yeast infections are common and are accompanied by itching and discharge.

Candida albicans infections are common following the use of antibiotic drugs, and may occur with use of birth control pills, consumption of sugar and refined carbohydrates, nutritional deficiencies, improper hygiene, allergies, and pregnancy.

What to do:

* Eat no sugar or refined carbohydrates. Simple sugars weakens the immune system and feeds yeast. Some individuals may wish to also avoid fruit and fruit juices which contain natural sugars.

* Avoid foods and supplements containing yeast.

* Supplement Lactobacillus acidophilus to restore normal intestinal flora.

* Eat fermented foods containing Lactobacillus

295

acidophilus:

> **Yogurt**
> **Kefir cheese**
> **Buttermilk**

* Avoid all other dairy products.

* Apply hydrogen peroxide solution (3 percent) topically.

* Supplement vitamin C up to bowel tolerance level.

* Supplement colostrum to support the immune system and help normalize intestinal flora.

* Supplement garlic-pure cloves are the best.

* Aloe vera may be applied topically (gel-helps relieve itching), as a douche, and consumed internally (two ounces four times daily).

* Echinacea is an effective anti-fungal agent and has a number of other immune support properties as well.

Beneficial supplementation:

> Vitamin A: 25,000 one to two times daily
> B Complex: (yeast free) 25-50 mg one to two times daily
> Biotin:
> Vitamin C: Up to bowel tolerance
> Vitamin E: 400-800 IU daily
> Tea Tree Oil: (topical) especially beneficial for nail fungus and as a douche
> Garlic:
> Colostrum: Two capsules two to four times daily
> Lactobacillus acidophilus: One to two capsules four to six times daily. Capsules may also be used as a suppository.
> **Herbs:** Echinacea, Garlic

How to avoid:

> Avoid antibiotics.
> Avoid sugar.
> Maintain health of the immune system with proper rest, diet, and exercise.
> Avoid stress.

Appendix I:

Castor Oil Pack

Successful applications of castor oil have been recorded in disturbances of the digestive system including the stomach, intestinal or colon problems; kidney, liver or gall bladder problems; disturbances of the lymphatic system; urinary and excretory systems; circulatory system; and some aspects of the nervous system.

Instructions for use of castor oil packs:

1. Prepare a soft flannel cloth folded two to three times thick. When folded it should be large enough to cover the entire area it is to be applied upon. For example, 8 x 12 inches for abdominal applications.

2. Pour the castor oil in a pan and soak the cloth in the oil. Wring out the excess oil so it is not dripping wet.

3. Apply the cloth to the area on the body requiring treatment. (Bedding should be protected in some way to prevent soiling.) Cover the oil-soaked cloth with a plastic covering and then place a heating pad on the top. Begin the heat setting at medium and increase it to high if it can be tolerated. It may be helpful to wrap a towel around the entire area. The pack should remain in place between one and 1 and 1/2 hours.

4. Frequency of use depends on individual situations. You may apply the castor oil packs (before retiring) in periods of three consecutive days with a couple of days in between. Continue this pattern until results are seen. Another recommendation is to apply the pack every other evening at bedtime for 10 or more applications.

5. Lukewarm soda water can be used to cleanse the area afterwards if desired.

6. The flannel pack can be stored in the pan for future use.

Vitamin C
Bowel Tolerance Level

To determine the optimal amount of vitamin C one needs at a particular time, Bowel Tolerance Level has shown to be the most effective.

Dr. Robert Cathcart III of Los Altos, CA, an infectious disease specialist who has had a great deal of experience and success with vitamin C, makes it his practice to establish for each of his patients their bowel-tolerance intake of vitamin C. This is the amount of vitamin C taken by mouth that is a little less than the amount that has a troublesome laxative effect. Cathcart found that vitamin C is most effective as an adjunct to appropriate conventional therapy, when needed, if it is ingested at the bowel-tolerance intake.

Bowel-tolerance levels vary from individual to individual and vary for the same individual at different times. Cathcart noted that the bowel-tolerance intake is usually very large for an individual who is seriously ill and becomes smaller as the individuals health improves. For a severely ill person, the bowel-tolerance limit may be more than 200 grams per day. Within a few days, as the condition is controlled, the limit may fall toward normal, 4 to 15 grams per day.

Cathcart has stated that vitamin C has little effect on acute symptoms until doses of 80-90 percent of bowel tolerance are reached.

Appendix III:
Formulas for Health
Courtesy of Great Life Labs, for more information call 1-800-526-4240

The following examples of nutritional supplement formulas may be of value when you are looking for specific nutritional support. Remember only your physician can diagnose or treat a medical condition. Check with your doctor about altering your nutritional intake.

AGING AND POOR ENERGY
Choline ....150 mg
Vitamin E...15 IU
PABA...100mg
Folic Acid ....40 mcg
Thiamin HCL..10 mg
Pantothenic Acid ....20 mg
Magnesium ....25 mg
RNA ....15 mg
Ascorbic Acid (Vitamin C) ....60 mg
Niacinamide ....25 mg
Vitamin B-6 ....10 mg
Vitamin B-12...5 mg
Inositol..40 mg
Biotin..150 mcg
Iodine..150 mcg
Zinc ....15 mg

CIRCULATION
Niacinamide ....202 mg
Niacin ....15 mg
Vitamin C...50 mg
Vitamin B-1 ....2. mg
Vitamin B-2 ....2.5 mg
Vitamin B-6 ....10 mg
Zinc ....2 mg
Vitamin B-12...2 mcg
    In a base of betaine HCL, manganese, citrus
    bioflavonoid, torula yeast, and alfalfa seed meal.

DIGESTIVE PROBLEMS
Vitamin B-1 ....2 mg
Vitamin B-2 ....2 mg
Niacinamide ....5 mg
Pancreas*...225 mg
Ox Bile ....30 mg
Papain..120 mg
Duodenum ....20 mg
Liver..20 mg
Betaine HCL...10 mg
Bromelain ....20 mg
    * Whole dried pancreas as a source of pancreatin,
    trypsin, amylase, lipase, lisotozyme, diastase, and
    chymosin.

ARTHRITIS

Vitamin A .... 5,000 IU
Vitamin C .... 150 mg
Niacin .... 6 mg
Niacinamide .... 570 mg
Calcium (citrus juice complex) .... 6 mg
Vitamin D .... 195 IU
Vitamin E .... 21 IU
Vitamin B-6 .... 6 mg
Vitamin B-12 .... 6 mcg
Magnesium (oxide, gluconate,
and citrus juice complex) .... 312 mg
Zinc .... 15 mg
Copper .... 750 mcg
Biotin .... 30 mcg
Pantothenic Acid .... 28 mg
> Cereal grass concentrate base containing lecithin, yeast, betaine HCL, RNA, PABA, potassium, and selenium.

SKIN (Rashes, sun sensitivity, etc.)

Vitamin A .... 3000 IU
Vitamin C .... 300 mg
Vitamin B1 .... 10 mg
Riboflavin .... 4 mg
Niacinamide .... 5 mg
Calcium .... 100 mg
Vitamin E 100IU
Folic Acid .... 100 mcg
Vitamin B12 .... 5 mcg
Magnesium .... 50 mg
Zinc .... 22 mg
Pantothenic Acid .... 100 mg
Beta Carotene .... 9000 mg
PABA .... 500 mg
RNA .... 15 mg
Selenium .... 60 mcg
Potassium .... 25 mg
Manganese .... 15 mg
Lysine .... 130 mg
> In a base of primrose oil, aloe vera, yucca, betaine and glutamic acid HCL, papain, oatstraw, horsetail, bee pollen and echinacea.

IMMUNITY (Frequent colds, sinusitis, post nasal drip, etc.)

Vitamin A .... 10,000 USP Units
Vitamin C .... 200 mg
Vitamin B-12 .... 2.5 mg
Pantothenic Acid .... 7 mg
Calcium .... 60 mg
Zinc .... 9.2 mg
Lemon Bioflavonoid Complex .... 30 mg
Thymus .... 25 mg
> In a base of rose hips, wheat germ oil, chlorophyll, lymph, and fermentation extract.

300

STRESS

Niacinamide	200 mg
Vitamin C	250 mg
Pantothenic Acid (B5)	40 mg
Vitamin B1	15 mg
Beta Carotene	1500 IU
Potassium	15 mg
Magnesium	100 g
Calcium	150 mg
Riboflavin (B2)	5 mg
Vitamin B12)	50 mcg
Vitamin B6	10 mg
Betaine Hydrochloride	10 mg

In a base of valerian root, comfrey root, chamomile, echinacea, raw adrenal concentrate, hops, aniseed & peppermint.

ENERGY AND IMMUNITY *(Especially for those over 35)*

Choline	212 mg
PABA	150mg
Vitamin E	22.50 mg
Methionine	75 mg
Folic Acid	600 mcg
Vitamin B1	15 mg
Pantothenic Acid (B5)	30 mg
Magnesium	38 mg
RNA	23 mg
Vitamin C	120 mg
Sodium Phosphate	0.75 mg
Brewers Yeast	75 mg
Vitamin B2	15 mg
Niacinamide	38 mg
Vitamin B6	15 mg
Vitamin B12	80 mcg
Inositol	60 mg
Biotin	230 mcg
Iodide	0.23 mg
Zinc	23 mg
Selenium	10 mcg
Beta Carotene	1250 IU
SOD	20 IU
Liver Extract	2 mg
Calcium	60 mg

In a base containing rose hips, alfalfa, raw pancreas, I-serine, L-cysteine and protein amino acid complex.

LIVER SUPPORT *(Detoxification)*

DL-Methionione............................200 mg
Choline Bitartrate...........................100 mg
Inositol..100 mg
Dandelion Root ....100 mg
Silymarin
Raw Liver Concentrate
  In a base of black radish, beet root powder, alfalfa, golden seal and rose hips

HYPOGLYCEMIA *(Low Blood Sugar)*

Vitamin A.....................................8000 IU
Vitamin B1...................................20 mg
Vitamin B2...................................20 mg
Niacinamide ....360 mg
Pantothenic Acid (B5).....................133 mg
Vitamin B6...................................60 mg
Vitamin B12.................................100 mcg
Inositol..80 mg
Biotin...300 mcg
Vitamin C.....................................1,000 mg
Vitamin E.....................................30 IU
Folic Acid ....800 mcg
PABA..50 mg
Calcium ....400 mg
Magnesium ....50 mg
Manganese...................................40 mg
Iodine...300 mcg
Chromium....................................333 mcg
Zinc ....30 mg
Choline ....424 mg
  In a base of raw pancreas, raw adrenal, liver concentrate, papain, bromelain, betaine HCL, sodium phosphate, methionine, chamomile, peppermint, comfrey, sarsparilla, dandelion, skullcap, alfalfa, and rosehips.

THYROID SUPPORT *(Weight Loss/Sluggish Metabolism)*

Atractylode rhizome.......................175mg
Polygonum multiforum....................175mg
Cuscuta semem 175mg
Cinnamon cortex...........................175mg
Siberian ginseng............................175mg
Astragalus radix............................175mg
Schisandra fructus.........................175mg
Psoralea semem 175mg
Crataegus fructus 175mg
Kelp 175mg
Asparagus radix 175mg
Colx semem..................................175mg
Tryrosine.....................................25,000 mcg
Raw adrenal, pituitary and liver
Rose hips

302

BIBLIOGRAPHY

All One People, (1990) Nutritech, Santa Barbara, CA

Airola, Paavo. *Hypoglycemia: A Better Approach* (1977) Health Plus Publishers, Phoenix, AZ.

American Heart Association *"The American Heart Association Diet* (1985) Dallas, TX.

Atkins, Robert. *Dr. Atkins' Nutritional Breakthrough-How To Treat Your Medical Condition Without Drugs* (1979) Bantam Books, New York, NY.

Atkins, Robert and Shirley Linde. *Dr. Atkins' Super Energy Diet* (1977) Bantam Books, New York, NY.

Bogert, Jean and Mame Porter. *Dietetics Simplified* (1937) The Macmillian Company, New York, NY.

Braggs, Paul. and Patricia Braggs. *The Shocking Truth About Water* (1985) Health Science, Santa Barbara, CA.

Bricklin, Mark. *Natural Healing* (1976) Rodale Press, Inc., Emmaus, PA.

Bureau of the Census, U.S. Department of Commerce, *Statistical Abstract of the United States* (1987) 107rd Edition.

Cook, William G. *The Yeast Connection* (1986) Professional Books, Jackson, TN.

Christian, Janet and Janet Greger. *Nutrition For Living* (1985) Benjamin/Cummings Publishing Co. Inc., Melno Park, CA.

Christopher, John R. *School of Natural Healing* (1976) Christopher Publications, Inc., Springville, UT.

Davis, Adelle. *Let's Eat Right to Keep Fit* (1970) New American Library, Inc. New York, NY.

Dunne, Lavon. *Nutrition Almanac* (1990) McGraw-Hill Publishing Company, New York, NY.

Eck, Paul. "How Increasing Your Energy Enhances Your Health, Emotions, Personality, and Your Ability to Achieve Success and Happiness" (1981) Healthview Newsletter, No. 27-29. The Eck Institute, Phoenix, AZ.

Eck, Paul and Beth Ley. *Dr. Paul Eck on Stress and Your Adrenal Glands* (1990) Christopher Lawrence Communications, Fargo, ND.

Erasmus, Udo. *Fats and Oils* (1986) Alive Books, Vancouver, British Columbia, Canada.

Gerson, Max. *A Cancer Therapy-Results of Fifty Cases- And The Cure of Advanced Cancer By Diet Therapy* (1985) Gerson Institute, Bonita, CA.

Gillen-Hansen, Peggy, and Bernd Friedlander. *It's Never Too Late!* (1990) Broadway Marketing, Fargo, ND.

Hafen, Brent. *First Aid for Health Emergencies* (1981) West Publishing Co. St. Paul, MN.

Hamilton, Eva May Nunnelley, Eleanor Noss Whitney, and Frances Sienkiewicz Sizer. *Nutrition, Concepts and Controversies* Third Edition (1979) West Publishing Company, St. Paul, MN.

Health and Wellness Confidential (1988) Boardroom Reports, Inc, New York, NY.

Hoffman, David. *The Herbal Handbook* (1988) Healing Arts Press, Rochester, VT.

Howell, Edward. *Enzyme Nutrition, The Food Enzyme Concept* (1985) Avery Publishing Group Inc., Wayne, NJ.

Kloss, Jethro. *Back to Eden* (1988) Back to Eden Publishing Co. Loma Linda, CA.

Langer, Stephen. *Solved: The Riddle of Illness* (1984) Keats Publishing, Inc., New Canaan, CT.

Leung, Albert. *Chinese Herbal Remedies* (1984) Universe Books, New York, NY.

Ley, Beth. *Colostrum: Nature's Gift to the Immune System* (1990) BL Publications, Fargo, ND.

Lineback, David and George Inglett. *Food Carbohydrates* (1982) The AVI Publishing Company Inc., Westport, CT.

Litt, Jerome. *Your Skin from Acne to Zits* (1989) Dembner Books, New York, NY.

Lorenzani, Shirley. *Candida: A Twentieth Disease* (1986) Keats Publishing, Inc., New Canaan, CT.

Lubecki, John. *Living Without Pain* (1985) Fair Oaks, CA.

Malinow, M.R. et al. "Alfafa" *American Journal of Clinical Nutrition,* (1979) 1,810-1,812.

304

McGarey, William. *Edgar Cayce and the Palma Christi* (1970) Edgar Cayce Foundation, Virginia Beach, VA.

McGarey, William. *The Edgar Cayce Remedies* (1983) Bantam Books, New York, NY.

Mensink, Ronald P. and Martijin B. Katan, "Effect of Dietary Trans-fatty Acids on High Density and Low Density Lipoprotein Cholesterol Levels in Healthy Subjects," *New England Journal of Medicine* (16 Aug 1990) *323 (7)*: 439-445

Mindell, Earl. *Vitamin Bible* (1979) Warner Books, New York, NY.

Mindell, Earl. *Unsafe at Any Meal* (1987) Warner Books, Inc. New York, NY.

The Mosby Medical Encyclopedia (1985) C.V. Mosby Company, New York, NY.

Neuman, Emil. *Health Tips* (1989) United Research Publishers, Leucadia, CA.

Newbold, H.L. *Mega Nutrients for Your Nerves* (1975) Berkley Books, New York. NY.

Null, Gary. *The Complete Guide to Health and Nutrition* (1984) Dell Publishing New York, NY.

Pauling, Linus. *How to Live Longer and Feel Better* (1986) Avon Books, New York, NY.

Pauling, Linus. *Vitamin C and Common Cold and Flu* (1976) W.H. Freeman and Company, San Francisco, CA.

Pfeifer, Carl. *Nutrition and Mental Ilness* (1987) Healing Arts Press, Rochester, Vermont

Philpott, William H., and Dwight K. Kalita. *Brain Allergies* (1980) Keats Publishing, Inc. New Canaan, CT.

Pritikin, Nathan and Patrick M. McGrady, Jr. *The Pritikin Program for Diet and Exercise* (1979) Bantam Books, Inc. New York, NY.

Rodale, J.I. *The Complete Book of Vitamins* (1975) Rodale Books, Inc., Emmaus, PA.

Roehrig, Karla. *Carbohydrate Biochemistry and Metabolism* (1984) The AVI Publishing Company, Inc. Westport, CT.

Royal, Penny C. *Herbally Yours* (1982) Sound Nutrition, Provo, UT.

Salaman, Maureen. *Foods That Heal* (1989) Statford Publishing, Melno Park, CA.

Selye, Hans. "The General Adaptation Syndrome and the Diseases and The Diseases of Adaptation" (February, 1946) *The Journal of Clinical Endocrinology, Vol. 6 (2).*

Shannon, Ira L. *Brand Name Guide to Sugar* (1977) Nelson-Hall Publishing, Chicago, ILL.

Stone, Irwin. *The Healing Factor: Vitamin C Against Disease* (1972) Putnam Publishing Group, New York, NY.

Susser, Arnold. *The Indigestion of America From Headaches to Hemorrhoids* (1987) Nutrition Society of America, Westfield, NJ.

Tenney, Louise. *Health Handbook* (1987) Woodland Books, Provo UT.

Tierra, Michael, *Planetary Herbology* (1988) Lotus Press, Santa Fe, NM.

Tortora, Gerard and Nicholas Anagnostakos, *Principles of Anatomy and Physiology* Third Edition, (1981) Harper and Row, New York, NY.

Trattler, Ross. Better *Health Through Natural Healing* (1985) McGraw-Hill Book Company, New York, NY.

Treben, Maria. *Health Through God's Pharmacy* (1980) Wilhelm Ennsthaler, Steyr, Austria.

United States Environmental Protection Agency: "Preliminary Assessment of Suspected Carcinogens in Drinking Water" (1975) Report to Congress, Washington, D.C.

Vitale, Joseph, and Selwyn Broitman. *Advances in Human Clinical Nutrition* (1982) John Wright PSG Inc. Boston, MA.

The Vitamin Herb Guide (1987) Global Health Ltd., Tofield, Alberta, Canada.

Wade, Carlson. *Amino Acids Book* (1985) Keat's Publishing, Inc. New Canaan, CT.

Webster, James. *Vitamin C: The Protective Vitamin* (1972) Universal-Award House, Inc., New York, NY.

Weil, Andrew. Natural Health, *Natural Medicine* (1990) Houghton Mifflin Company, Boston, MA.

INDEX

309

311

312

315

317

HOW DID WE GET SO **FAT?**

by Dr. Arnold J. Susser and Beth M. Ley

A guide for those who want to safely obtain their weight goals without going crazy

Leading U.S. medical authorities consider obesity to be our most widespread nutritional disorder. An estimated 100 million Americans are currently obese. We spent an estimated 33 billion dollars on diets and diet-related products last year. **And we are _Still Fat!_** Take a look at the foods you are eating, your eating habits. How much refined sugar do you eat How much fiber? Do you eat processed foods? Partially hydrogenated or hydrogenated oils? Margarine? Fried food? Do you stuff yourself to the point of discomfort?

Find out why these questions are so important to your waistline from one of the nation's leading nutritionists, **Dr. Arnold J. Susser, R.P., Ph.D.**, and nutrition writer Beth Ley, in *How Did We Get So Fat?* Lose weight easily, safely, and permanently...*without dieting!* Learn about dangerous and bogus diet supplements and learn about one's that work.

96 pages, 1994 paper back.

Suggested retail: **$7.95** *(ISBN 0-9642703-0-7)*

Health Learning Handbook Series:

Health Learning Handbooks by Beth M. Ley are designed to provide useful and interesting information about ways to improve one's health and well-being. Education about what good health is and what the body needs to obtain and maintain good health is of critical importance so that we can make the best informed decisions about our health. Health Learning Handbooks are an easy to read, valuable addition to your bookshelf!

Castor Oil : Its Healing Properties

Castor Oil and Its Healing Properties is an easy to read educational guide explaining the applications of castor oil including warts, liver or age spots, papillomas, pigmented moles, body ulcers, slow-to-heal umbilicus of a newborn infant, eye irritations, lack of proper growth of hair in little children, to stimulate growth of eyelashes or eyebrows, to relieve aching feet, to soften corns and calluses and much more! The book includes complete instructions for use of castor oil packs and features an interview with Dr. William McGarey, Director of the A.R.E. Clinic in Phoenix, AZ.

Sug Retail: $3.95

Dr. John Willard on Catalyst Altered Water

Dr. John Willard on Catalyst Altered Water features exclusive interviews with the creator and patent holder of the amazing Catalyst Altered Water (known as Willard Water), Dr. Willard, Sr., Professor Emeritus of Chemistry at the S.D. School of Mines and Technology. The book summarizes the research and experience showing the potential Willard Water has to offer to improve the well-being of plants, animals, and humans. The book, a vital tool for all users of Willard Water, is a must for best results!

Sug. Retail: $3.95

Colostrum:
Nature's Gift to the Immune System

Colostrum: Nature's Gift to the Immune System, explains why immunity is so important to our health and well-being and offers suggestions on how we can naturally support our immune system. In this book you will learn what colostrum is, find out why colostrum can benefit the immune system of people of all ages, and read about the scientific research supporting the supplemental use of colostrum and its benefits. In addition, this book provides valuable information about AIDS, its signs and symptoms, and about how the AIDS virus destroys the immune system. This book features an exclusive interview with a well-known, prestigious medical doctor and author, Dr. Keith W. Sehnert.

Sug. Retail: $3.95